Physicochemical Anthropology
Part I: Human Behavioral Structure

Physicochemical Anthropology

Part I: Human Behavioral Structure

Norman R. Joseph

University of Illinois at the Medical Center, Chicago, Ill.

1 figure and 3 tables, 1978

S. Karger · Basel · München · Paris · London · New York · Sydney

By the same author

Comparative Physical Biology
X + 234 p., 7 fig., 45 tab., 1973
ISBN 3−8055−1485−9

Cataloging in Publication
Joseph, Norman R.
Physicochemical anthropology / Norman R. Joseph. − Basel; New York: Karger, 1978
Contents: pt. 1. Human behavioral structure.
1. Anthropology 2. Chemistry, Physical I. Title
GN 24 J83p
ISBN 3−8055−2793−4

© Copyright 1978 by S. Karger AG, 4011 Basel (Switzerland), Arnold-Böcklin-Strasse 25
Printed in Switzerland by Thür AG Offsetdruck, Pratteln
ISBN 3−8055−2793−4

Contents

Contents

Preface

A theoretical conceptual scheme is required for the structure and organization of any physicochemical or biological science to have any general validity; such a scheme requires an absolutely sound system of successive approximations. The most important of these is the 'first approximation', or basic presupposition. Unless this is absolutely unquestionable, all subsequent approximations carry a residue of uncertainty, with the ever-present possibility of serious or fatal errors. Thus, the first step of constructing a sound theoretical scheme must be an act of doubt or absolute skepticism. This was the fundamental step in *Descartes'* method. The principle retains its validity throughout subsequent periods, including the 20th century, as shown by *Husserl* (1970) in his *Cartesian Meditations*.

In the conceptual scheme of Physicochemical Anthropology, as developed in the following pages, the first approximation, or basic presupposition, is the absolute certainty of the existence of the human race as a Linnaean taxonomic species, recognized as *Homo sapiens*. To doubt this is to suppose that all human life and experience is a pure subjective illusion. This is a doctrine of 'solipsism', which no one seriously believes.

Then anthropology may be defined as the science of man. One of its main branches can be defined, as in the present volume, as physicochemical anthropology, which is based on the absolute preconception that any individual man or woman is a living organism, and that his structure and behavior depend on the structure and behavior of living protoplasm (*Huxley*, 1868). This has been accepted by all competent anatomists, histologists, and morphologists since the time of *Purkinje, Schleiden, Schwann* and *von Helmholtz*, dating from the first half of the 19th century.

The foregoing preconception can then be stated that anthropology or the science of man must include as one of its foundations the subject of the physical chemistry, reactivity and behavior of protoplasm, considered as a heterogeneous *structured* physicochemical system. If this is accepted as a first approximation, then it is necessary to rule out any conceptual scheme that treats protoplasm as an intracellular *solution*, or perfect mixture of colloids, water and inorganic electrolytes. This must be distinguished from a heterogeneous system consisting of partially miscible lyophilic colloids. Thus, we must distinguish between a theory of 'heterogeneous substances', as developed by *J. W. Gibbs* (1875–1928) and a special case of this known as the 'Donnan equilibrium' (1911), or 'theory of membrane equilibrium and membrane potentials in the presence of a non-dialyzable electrolyte'. Unfortunately, these two theories have been confused by later generations of biochemists, physiologists, and morphologists under the misleading term, 'the Gibbs-Donnan equilibrium'. This is an error which has led to a false negative first approximation in the present theory of 'active transport', which assumes that water-electrolyte distribution cannot be explained by Gibbs' 'equilibrium of heterogeneous substances'. This error results from the presupposition that cells and tissues are unstructured, homogeneous phases contained within systems of semi-permeable membranes. This leads to the serious fallacy, pointed out by Fischer and Hooker (1933) that water-electrolyte balance is not subject to the general thermodynamics of heterogeneous systems, but that it requires special forms of metabolic energy. These are not referred to the general nature of heterogeneous structured lyophilic colloidal systems.

The theory of so-called 'active transport' developed since the work of Fischer and Hooker has failed to correct the fundamental fallacy which they pointed out. Hence the entire fabric of subsequent theories of active transport and metabolic control of water-electrolyte balance is open to serious doubt and skepticism. Thus, no theory of physicochemical anthropology can be based on the absolute preconceptions of active transport or intracellular respiratory metabolism. As will be shown in the following, any valid theory requires a general theory of protoplasmic structure and behavior. This problem is discussed in chapter 1 of the following, under the subject of Structuralism. This includes a discussion of the lyotropic series of Hofmeister (1888), which antedates by a period of nearly 50 years the work of Fischer and Hooker on the lyophilic colloids. This, as based on Carnot's principle, Gibbs' phase rule, and the general physiology of Claude Bernard, was the basis of a conceptual scheme for comparative physical biology (Joseph, 1973).

There are inaccessible states in the neighborhood of any given state.

Carnot's principle

The stability of the milieu intérieur is the primary condition for freedom and independence of existence.   Claude Bernard

Chapter 1

Structuralism

Any physicochemical system at any specified temperature or pressure is characterized not only by its chemical composition, but also by its *structure*. At ordinary temperatures but at any pressure higher than that of a perfect vacuum, the most unstructured systems are represented by pure gases. When a given kind of atom or molecule in the vapor state is surrounded by only a few other similar particles, it is subject to very infrequent molecular collisions, and for relatively long intervals of time is separated by rather great distances from other atoms and molecules. However, in any containing vessel, it has a certain calculable or measurable kinetic energy that is proportional to the absolute temperature.

Therefore, depending on the magnitude of the enclosed volume, it undergoes numerous elastic collisions with the walls of the vessel. At extremely small distances from any elastic walls, it is subject to certain forces of attraction or repulsion. The attractive forces include a group known as the *'van der Waals'* attractions, and include 'dipole-dipole' and 'dipole-induced dipole' attractions that operate at very short distances. Also, at such distances, there occur the 'London dispersion forces' that depend on oscillating electrical charges between any given pairs of atoms and molecules. These are partly responsible, with other physical and chemical forces, for adsorption of atoms or molecules at the surface of the walls. Finally, at extremely short distances, there are repulsive forces between atomic nuclei that are responsible for the elastic collisions that repel the gas particles from the walls.

All these forces of attraction or repulsion are inherent in each individual atom or molecule even when it is relatively isolated from all other particles, as in a state of high vacuum. Thus, each particle is characterized by its known mass, and also by its kinetic and potential energy. The kind of atom or molecule, helium, neon, hydrogen, or nitrogen, is a property that describes its 'firstness'. This refers to the atomic or molecular species: H_2, He, Ne, N_2, O_2, and so forth. The energy, kinetic or potential, is a coordinated property belonging generally to a class denoted as 'secondness'. Finally, a third kind of property depending on the trajectory of a given particle or group of particles extended over a long period of time is called the 'thirdness' of any such group of atoms or molecules. It is a statistical property that depends on the coordinates q, and the momenta p, of each particle in a statistical *ensemble*, integrated over a definite period of time. It is described by what is known as a phase integral in 'statistical mechanics' (*Gibbs*, 1901). Thus, the infinitesimal dp dq denotes an element of phase space; the phase integral is defined as $\int D\,dp\,dq$.

Density in Phase

In a dynamical system of particles characterized as above by the individual values of the coordinates q and the momenta p, the generalized velocity of any particle $\dot q$ is related to the total energy H, where:

$$H = T + V,$$

where T is the total kinetic energy, and V is the potential energy of the system. If a large number of such systems is considered, the differential:

$$dp_1 \ldots dp_n\,dq_1 \ldots dq_n,$$

may be defined as an element of *extension in phase* (*Gibbs*, 1901). Here, n denotes the total number of particles in a given ensemble, whereas p and q refer to the generalized momenta and coordinates, as they vary over any period of time. The generalized motion is then described, within certain restrictions, by the phase integral, as described above. In that expression, dp dq denotes an element of extension in phase, and D denotes the 'density in phase', referring to the relative probability of any given system occurring in a given region of phase space. In general, for any given ensemble of n molecules or particles in a gas phase, the probability of uniform distribution is extremely high, and the system may be said to be unstructured.

In the case of liquids and solids, the function D is very high as compared to its value in a coexistent vapor phase. Thus, in the case of water, the vapor pressure at 100 °C is 1 atmosphere, and the molal volume is:

$$22.4 \times 373/273 = 30.2 \text{ liters.}$$

At the same temperature and pressure, the molal volume of liquid water is about 18 ml or 0.018 liters. Therefore, the relative values of density in phase are in the ratio:

$$\frac{D_l}{D_g} = \frac{30.2}{0.018} = 55.51 \times 30.2 = 1,676,$$

where D_l and D_g refer respectively to the liquid and gas phase.

Therefore, over a time interval of 1,676 sec, a given water molecule spends on the average only 1 sec in the vapor phase and 1,675 sec in the liquid phase (for a closed system in reversible equilibrium). In such systems, liquid and solid phases are regarded as *condensed* and of *low entropy*. The vapor phase or steam is disorganized, unstructured, and of high entropy.

Thus, physicochemical systems in relation to physicochemical state must be characterized not only by chemical composition, but also by order, disorder, and *structure*. Chemical composition and structure are properties of 'firstness'. Energy, entropy, order, and disorder are aspects of 'secondness'. Extension of firstness and secondness over long periods of time may be represented in the form of phase integrals. In any case, a phase integral would exhibit a property of 'thirdness', or the evolutionary history of any physicochemical system representing the elements of extension and density in phase. Thus, the concept of 'structuralism' should be understood as a dynamic concept of evolutionary structure in time.

Anthropological Structuralism

In the science of anthropology, 'firstness' is represented by man, regarded as a species of primate known as *'homo sapiens'*. Physical anthropology may be regarded as the study of human anatomy of the various races of man at various stages of their histories and phylogenetic development, studied both as living and fossilized forms. This would include the chemical and structural study of the morphology of human protoplasm, as represented by the various kinds of cells and tissues of the human body.

The functions of the neuromuscular system, sense organs and brain are aspects of the 'secondness' of anatomical, histological, and morphological structures. 'Secondness' is related to 'firstness' as function and behavior are related to anatomy and morphology. Both firstness and secondness develop in a space time continuum of phylogeny, ontogeny and geographical distribution. These are aspects of cultural and philosophical anthropology (chapter 11). Cultural and philosophical anthropology depend on language, both spoken and written, or other forms of communication, on the development of literature, science, and philosophical thought. Development of these fields requires prolonged experience, and extension in time of the properties of firstness and secondness. In addition to the development of agriculture and technology, advanced cultures observe the 'pursuit of happiness' or the principle of 'agapism' or 'evolutionary love'. All human societies beyond the primitive paleolithic level have cultivated to a certain extent philosophical or humanistic studies, although these may have been confined to small groups of a privileged elite. All such studies and disciplines require the qualities of 'thirdness' extended over prolonged periods of time embracing the life experience of many generations. The subjects of philosophical and cultural anthropology are concerned with thought, the pursuit of happiness, the principles of reason, the art of living, and the cultivation of agapism or evolutionary love. These aspects of thirdness presuppose elementary security in the continuation or preservation of firstness and secondness, or the functions of survival and reproduction (chapter 11).

Protoplasm: Firstness and Secondness

Since the early years of the 19th century, protoplasm has been recognized as a biological and chemical entity. The word is derived from the Greek 'protos' (first) and 'plasma' (formed substance) and is used to denote the 'first formed substance' of the plant or animal cellular structure. As commonly used, it refers to the hard, slimy, heterogeneous colloidal substance characteristic of intracellular substances in general, whether plant or animal. Well-directed studies of the physicochemical and morphological characteristics of protoplasm can thus be dated from about 1840, the approximate date of the 'cell theory' of *Schleiden* and *Schwann*. Since that time, histologists, histochemists and other students of the phenomena of life have generally recognized that 'irritability' of living matter is intimately related to the physicochemical responsiveness of living cells and tissues (*Peirce*, 1878, 1892).

Two main classes of intracellular macromolecules have been generally recognized — nuclear or cytoplasmic. These are physically separable and microscopically heterogeneous. They are identifiable by various methods of optical and X-ray spectroscopy, and by the methods of electron microscopy. Theoretical and experimental studies have shown that the molecular kinetic units of both cytoplasm and nuclei are extremely high, of the order of several millions. Thus, the molecular weights of intracellular macromolecules are of higher orders of magnitude than those of such typical soluble extracellular proteins as the serum albumins or globulins, about 70,000—150,000, or of egg albumin, about 40,000 g/mole.

Preparations of these proteins never show the actual properties of truly living systems, such as irritability, contractility, or reproduction. With few exceptions (those of the filtrable viruses), these properties are confined to intracellular protoplasmic structures composed of heterogeneous colloidal systems of macromolecules, water, and mixtures of physiological ions. These properties, accordingly, cannot be duplicated in the phenomena of 'membrane equilibrium' or 'membrane potentials', as studied with *in vitro* preparations according to the methods of the '*Donnan* equilibrium' (*Donnan*, 1911). The reason for this is that the traditional models of 'membrane equilibrium' apply only to homogeneous solutions with the property of perfect mixing.

Physicochemical systems that are homogeneous and therefore perfectly mixed, show the property of being relatively unconstrained and of high entropy.

Heterogeneous systems of the same components are imperfectly mixed and partially or absolutely immiscible. They are therefore characterized by the property of low or negative entropy, and systems have the property of high configurational free energy. According to classical or reversible thermodynamics:

$$\Delta G = \Delta H - T\Delta S,$$

where ΔG is the free energy of mixing the given phases. ΔH is the corresponding change of enthalpy, or heat of mixing, and ΔS is the corresponding change of entropy. A stable heterogeneous system requires a positive value of ΔG. If the system is *athermal* (stable with respect to temperature), ΔH is zero, and $T\Delta S$ is negative. This implies that mixing, or the tendency to form homogeneous solutions, is attended by an increase of free energy. Hence spontaneous mixing of intracellular or nuclear phases cannot occur in the stable or invariant standard state. This means that all such stable heterogeneous systems are supplied with negative entropy or positive configurational free energy.

It follows that the firstness of protoplasm may be defined as its composition with respect to macromolecular polyelectrolytes, water, and the characteristic electrolytes. Its secondness can then be described as the distribution of these substances between the various phases of the heterogeneous system, including both intracellular and extracellular phases. Distribution depends on 'negative entropy' and configurational free energy. This determines maximal work, isometric tensions, and irritability of any part of the neuromuscular system. These properties imply physiological functions and quantitative measures of physiological activity. Since these properties depend mainly on intracellular changes of state that involve water, they are also related to changes of respiratory metabolism, involving glycolysis, proteolysis, or lipolytic cleavage.

Thus, the firstness and secondness of the properties of protoplasm may be distinguished as follows:

Firstness	Secondness
Composition	
Proteins	dielectric constant
Nucleoproteins	hydration energy
Water	negative entropy
Electrolytes	configurational free energy
(NaCl, KCl,	work capacity
$CaCl_2$, $MgCl_2$)	isometric tension
Temperature	elasticity
Pressure	electrical potentials
	chemical potentials of water and inorganic electrolytes

Protoplasmic firstness is thus described by chemical composition, temperature, and pressure. Secondness is described by energies, entropies, and potentials, as they are related to the various physiological functions of irritability, contractility, and conduction. It now remains to describe the properties of 'thirdness', as they are related to the extension in time of firstness and secondness.

Extension in Time

In the 20th century, the normal human life expectancy is of the order of 70–80 years. This represents a continuous or 'synechistic' development from infancy to normal senescence. Such a life span represents only an infinitesimal fraction of the entire human experience extended over the entire anthropological life experience of billions of human beings over time intervals of the order of 1 or 2 million years *(Montague)*. Over this entire period, the anatomy, chemical morphology, and structure of human cells and tissues have been retained, developing according to laws of growth and mitosis for each of billions of individual lives. Physical anthropology is the science of human anatomy and morphology, as studied in living races of man, or in fossilized remains that date from paleozoic ages.

These studies represent the properties of 'firstness' extended over long periods of geological time. The properties of secondness, such as methods of locomotion, walking, climbing, swimming, and so forth, can only be inferred by hypothesis, relating to the constraints imposed by morphology. Thus, bipedal walking appears to have been preceded by quadrupedal locomotion in early forerunners of man. The anatomical changes were attended by changes in the size and shape of the skull, of the oral cavity, and of the dentition.

The development of speech and language can then be inferred to involve secondness and thirdness, as they have been extended over geological ages. Thus, all properties of human communication have evolved over periods of geological time, and may be regarded as examples of anthropological 'thirdness'.

The factors of anthropological evolution then include those of fortuitous chance ('tychism') and continuity of genes and protoplasm (continuity, 'holding together', or 'synechism'). Fortuitous chance is the basis of Darwinian 'natural selection', and synechism is the basis of Linnaean continuity and taxonomy. These are properties of firstness and secondness, as they imply morphology and behavior. However, as emphasized by *Peirce* (1878, 1892), a third principle (evolutionary love or 'agapism' must certainly have been operative in cultural and philosophical anthropology (chapter 11). This requires many generations of well-directed human experience involving thought, language, art, literature, recorded history, and science. These aspects of experience extended over many human generations belong to 'thirdness', as it is based on phylogeny and ontogeny. In addition to the elementary principles of chance and logic, it requires the operation of agapism or evolutionary love, applied over long epochs of human history. The principle of agapism, based on the human emotions of well-directed evolutionary love, is an essential element of human reason, which requires long-term purpose or qualities of 'thirdness' based on purposeful experience and value judgements.

Lability of Dielectric Energy

Protoplasm has long been recognized (since the 17th and 18th centuries) to possess in a high degree the property of irritability, and *Bernard* understood that biological reactivity always showed an 'organizing sense' inherent in protoplasm (chapter 8).

In the following chapters, it will be shown that this inherent organizing sense depends on the lability of intracellular colloidal aggregates in processes of disaggregation or 'Entmischung' (unmixing). In such processes, water becomes liberated from a hydrated or bound form ('ice-like') to a free liquid form, behaving as an aqueous solvent with the properties of a mixture rather than with those of a solid aggregate. In contraction or in the increase of isometric tension, the intracellular water of the myofibrils is calculated to pass from a standard state in which the dielectric constant is about 30 to a contracted state in which the disordered water is temporarily characterized by a dielectric constant of 80, resembling that of extracellular fluids (*Joseph*, 1973; *Catchpole and Joseph*, 1974). In this process, dielectric energy of the magnitude of about 80 cal/kg water is released. It is either converted quantitatively as external work, or it appears as heat in a process of isometric tension.

Muscular work and changes of tension are practically continuous processes in all normal human behavior. They are manifested in the processes of walking, talking, standing, sitting, and all other neuromuscular behavior. Every movement of the body implies some kind of redistribution of hydration energy and of configurational free energy within the body cells and tissues. Since these involve intracellular changes of state of water, they result in changes of solubilities of the various nutrients and metabolites, with consequent changes in the rates of anaerobic and aerobic respiratory metabolism.

All such processes depend on the lability of protoplasm in two or more possible states of aggregation. Together these consitute all the protoplasmic processes listed previously as aspects of 'secondness'. They include all changes of chemical potentials of water and electrolytes and the electrical potentials of all ions. Metabolic reactions and rates are aspects of 'secondness' rather than of 'firstness'. Thus, they depend on the lability of protoplasm and the states of the aqueous dielectric or dispersion medium. This is contrary to the views of contemporary physiologists and biochemists, who tend to regard glycolytic respiratory metabolism as primary, and distribution or transport as secondary. This view, as developed in the theory of 'active transport', is fundamentally fallacious, since it is based on the concept of homogeneous states of water within semipermeable membranes, and since it requires suspension or negation of the laws of thermodynamics (*Joseph*, 1973). These difficulties are avoided by assigning priority to the phylogenetic and ontogenetic 'firstness' of protoplasm as a living entity with the characteristics of labile states of dielectric and hydration energies. Thus, intermediary respiratory metabolism is classed by its secondness along with all other behavioral characteristics.

Lyotropic Energies

Crystalline solids of $NaCl$, KCl, $CaCl_2$, and other halides of the alkaline and alkaline earth metals are very soluble in water, which is a polar liquid of high dielectric constant. They are much less soluble in non-polar liquids of low dielectric constant, such as benzene, chloroform, or ethyl ether. Solubilities of crystalline electrolytes depend fundamentally on two kinds of attractive forces within the crystal lattice (or lattice energies, which tend to resist solubilization) and lyophilic energies or forces of attraction within the liquid solvent. When the solvent is water, this is called 'hydration energy'. In the following chapters, this is taken to depend not only on the inherent nature of water as a solvent, but also on its properties as an intracellular dispersion medium, forming solid or semisolid ('ice-like') aggregates with intracellular macromolecular aggregates. Thus, the composition of protoplasm with respect to its macromolecular components, water, and electrolytes is a property of 'firstness'. The lyotropic or hydrophilic properties of the ions depend on the nature of the dispersion medium, taken as a variable measure of 'secondness'.

It is then taken for granted that all measures of 'firstness' and 'secondness' are fundamental phylogenetic and ontogenetic functions of protoplasmic structure. Therefore, theories such as *Donnan*'s 'theory of membrane equilibrium and membrane potentials in the presence of a non-dialyzable electrolyte' are inadequate to explain the properties of living cells and tissues, because it takes no account of the conditions of firstness, secondness or thirdness of living protoplasm. *Gibbs*' 'equilibrium of heterogeneous substances' is far more general than any theory of membrane equilibrium, since it is valid for any possible states of aggregation, miscibility or immiscibility of any system of phases and components.

The free energy of hydration of any kind of inorganic ion depends on the ionic charge and radius, and on the dielectric constant of the solvent or dispersion medium (*Born*, 1920; *Laidler and Pegis*, 1957). The ionic radii can be determined from X-ray diffraction studies of the crystalline state, using the data of *Goldschmidt* (1926) and *Pauling* (1944). When the molal work of charging a system of ions in the vapor state is calculated theoretically, the following results are obtained (kcal/mole):

K	Na	Ca	Mg	Cl
123	164	615	824	90

These values *in vacuo* refer to a dielectric constant of 1.0. Applying a corrected value for the radius of the solvated ions in water, the corresponding values of the work terms are (kcal/mole):

K	Na	Ca	Mg	Cl
1.23	1.64	6.15	8.24	0.90

Hence the 'free energies of hydration', which represent the work of transferring 1 mole of any kind of ion from a vacuum to water are given by (kcal/mole):

K	Na	Ca	Mg	Cl
121.8	162.36	608.85	811.8	89.1

These values of hydration or lyotropic energies are found to be proportional to z_i^2/b_i, where z_i is the charge, and b_i is the ionic radius, estimated from the corrected values of the crystal radii.

The series:

Cl < K < Na < Ca < Mg,

was recognized by *Hofmeister* as early as 1888, and was denoted by protein chemists as the 'lyotropic series' or '*Hofmeister* series' of colloid chemistry (*Hofmeister*, 1888; *Loeb*, 1924). According to general physicochemical theory, the attractive or repulsive forces between colloidal particles and inorganic ions are reciprocal; the 'lyotropic series' is valid not only as criteria for the effects of colloids on the ions, but also for the related effects of the ions on the colloids (*Joseph*, 1935, 1936, 1938). It has been shown that many of the reciprocal forces between ions and protoplasm depend on the characteristic values of z_i^2/b_i for the various physiological ions (*Joseph*, 1971a, b; 1973).

These effects are exerted on the properties of 'firstness', including the lyotropic properties of the aqueous dispersion medium. Electrolyte distributions and potentials are then inherent properties of the ions and of the state of the intracellular dispersion medium. They do not depend on 'transport' phenomena, and are independent of intermediary metabolism and of membrane permeabilities.

Lyotropic energies depend on the nature of each kind of intracellular phase. Thus, in resting skeletal muscle, in which the dielectric constant is 30, the value of the free energies of hydration are (kcal/mole):

K	Na	Ca	Mg	Cl
3.28	4.38	6.56	8.76	2.41

Comparing these values with those for pure water (dielectric constant 80), we obtain hydration energies in muscle as referred to water or extracellular fluids (kcal/mole):

K	Na	Ca	Mg	Cl
2.05	2.74	10.25	13.7	1.41

It is seen that these values are likewise proportional to z_i^2/b_i, and that they conform to the position of each ion in the *Hofmeister* lyotropic series. Each value represents what will hereafter be described as the 'change of standard chemical potential' between an intracellular phase of protoplasm and an extracellular fluid. Denoted as $\Delta\mu_i^\circ$, it is a property of 'firstness'. However, in stimulated protoplasm, its value may approach zero. It thus represents a measure of cellular irritability or responsiveness, such as a change of work capacity or tension. The modified value of $\Delta\mu_i^\circ$ is then an aspect of 'secondness' or of protoplasmic lability or responsiveness. This is a measure of both firstness and secondness rather than of metabolism or respiration, which are likewise aspects of secondness. In such responses, secondness should always be referred to firstness, and never to other aspects of secondness, such as metabolism or permeability (*Joseph*, 1973). Dielectric, hydrophilic, and lyophilic properties represent the primary nature of intracellular colloidal aggregates. These are inherently reactive, irritable, and independent of metabolic controls (*Joseph*, 1973).

Physical Chemistry of Protoplasm

The primary function of protoplasm is to exist in the living cells and tissues of any given species. This implies in the human being the phylogeny of the species, of any given individual, and the ontogenetic development from birth to a given period of his curve of growth and development. Chemical morphology and histology at any time constitute the primary properties of the existent anatomical and protoplasmic structures. The characterization of given sets of cells and tissues as a physicochemical system is the first step necessary in determining the laws of structure, function, and behavior.

As a first approximation for any kind of protoplasmic structure it is necessary to determine its composition with respect to water and five kinds of ions (Na, K, Ca, Mg, and Cl). The remainder of the protoplasmic mass may then be estimated as grams of cellular material per kilogram water (*Joseph,* 1973).

By application of *Gibbs'* (1875, 1928) 'equilibrium of heterogeneous substances', the phase rule, and the principle of *Carnot-Clausius* (1824–1869), the following thermodynamic functions can then be determined or calculated: (1) the chemical potential of water, and (2) the equivalent change of chemical potential of each kind of ion, measured as $\Delta\mu_i/z_i$, where z_i is the ionic charge, taken as negative for anions.

Chapter 2

Cartesian Dualism

According to the principles of structuralism outlined in chapter 1, it is necessary to establish at least a dualistic relationship between the human mind and the human body, or between the human being at any time and his functions and behavior. Over an extended period of time, it is necessary to consider also the development of body and mind during periods of growth and aging. Hence, the threefold relations of mind, body, and time are the essentials of any consideration of the problem of 'Cartesian dualism'.

In *Descartes*' method, as set forth in his *Discourse on Method,* the first step in establishing his philosophical presuppositions is an act of absolute skepticism and doubt. He sets out to find first principles that are absolutely certain, and finds this certainty in his own existence. This is stated in the famous *cogito ergo sum.* Thus, 'firstness' is embodied in his own thought; this implies the certainty of his own existence.

Thus, in the Cartesian philosophy, thought was primary, matter and energy were primarily of a spatio-temporal relationship, and reasoning was primarily mathematical, subjective, *a priori,* and rationalist rather than empiricist. The reason for this is evident. Firstness, according to the Cartesian method, was thought or cogitation. From the beginning, he tended to regard life (or what since about 1840 would have been based on protoplasm) as the secondary principle of his dualism (or as 'secondness'). This was certainly rationalist, *a priori,* and reductionist. Like any other absolutist or non-empirical method of thinking, it produced abstractions later to be characterized by *James* (1912) for their 'thinness'. The proper classification of human protoplasm by the principle of anthropological firstness is to be found in a lecture by *Huxley* (1868) and in an essay by *Peirce* (1892): *Man's Glassy Essence.* In his essay, *Peirce* found that the reactivity of protoplasm (or its secondness) depended on its lyophilic or hydrophilic properties. This would necessarily imply processes of thought or cogitation as well as properties of neuromuscular behavior. The views of *Huxley* were essentially in agreement with this view of the 'firstness' of protoplasm.

In the subject of physicochemical anthropology, one begins by accepting the certainty of the existence of the human race, or of the Linnaean species, *homo sapiens.* Since the cell theory of *Schleiden and Schwann* (about 1840), and the early theories of *Purkinje, von Helmholtz,* and *von Mohl* of about the same period, it is possible to relate anthropology to the structure and behavior of human protoplasm. Thus, the phylogenetic existence of any human being, including that of *Descartes* himself, implies not only his existence (anatomical and morphological), but also his behavior, thought, and philosophy. These are functions of his time and place in history and of preceding or antecedent conditions of human thought and behavior up to his own time. Cartesian dualism, as a historical development, was a product of metaphysical questioning that continues to be of interest until our own time.

Chance and Logic

Descartes was unable to doubt his own existence. According to his method of reasoning, this included all essential attributes of material bodies, including the necessary properties of extension in space and time. These properties imply the physical concepts of motion, mechanical energy, and momentum. Hence, physical reality is necessarily dependent on the existence of material particles, in what *Newton* was to recognize as physical space and time.

Huxley's views of anthropology, as expressed in *Man's Place in Nature,* were essentially in agreement with the firstness of anatomy, morphology and protoplasmic reactivity, as of primary importance in human evolution. *Huxley* had the great advantage over *Descartes* of possessing well-defined views on anatomy, physiology, and on comparative zoology and phylogeny. On the contrary, *Descartes*' views were essentially those of a rationalist, *a priori* type of geometer, who fancied that his combination of the principles of algebra and geometry into the new science of analytical geometry could lead to the combination of all sciences by such *a priori* synthetic methods. The ultimate failure of *Descartes*' type of dualistic reasoning was to be found in its inadequacy in the field of physiology, medicine, and other branches of the biological sciences. This was due to the omission of the sense organs and the emotions from his conceptual scheme, which remained fundamentally *a priori*, geometrical and mechanistic.

The principle known by *Peirce* as 'agapism' or 'evolutionary love' was omitted from Cartesian dualism. The omission had the important advantage, greatly appreciated by physicists, mathematicians, chemists, and other students of the non-biological sciences of eliminating the interfering element of 'subjectivity' on the part of human observers, who can always be influenced by conscious or unconscious sources of bias. For this reason, introspective psychology, as understood by *William James,* has been criticized for its un-Cartesian non-geometrical subjectivity based on non-experimental value judgements. *James*' 'Pragmatism' and *Peirce*'s 'Pragmaticism' are frankly based on subjective value judgements of an empiricist nature. This has tended to antagonize or to alienate psychologists of the behaviorist school, who prefer quantitative physical measurements in human physiology to the more intangible judgements inherent in agapistic value judgements.

Neutral Monism and Reactive Dualism

Peirce, in considering the problem of Cartesian dualism, advanced three possible solutions of the problem:

(1) The firstness of the material parts of the body. This is a doctrine of 'materialism'.

(2) A doctrine of neutral monism, in which mind and body share equally in the relation of the individual to the external world. This is rejected in favor of:

(3) The view of 'objective idealism', in which our ideas of external reality originate in a real, non-subjective, external universe brought into a system of organized perceptions and concepts through sense organs, scientific instruments, communication, and empirical experience. This is the generally accepted method of the exact physical sciences, which attempt to eliminate the subjective aspects of neutral monism. There is no way of arriving at the principle of the 'firstness' of protoplasm, without the prior formulations of concepts such as the cell theory of *Schleiden and Schwann,* or of the observations of microscopists such as *Purkinje, von Mohl, von Helmholtz* or more recently of *Frey-Wyssling.* The observations lead to the principle of 'structuralism', which should not be mistaken for a principle of 'materialism'.

The concept either of materialism or of neutral monism would imply the 'firstness' of non-living protoplasm, of inorganic materials, or of lifeless substance.

On the contrary, according to the principles of structuralism, the reactivity of protoplasm in the living state implies its organization as a purposeful hetero-geneous colloidal aggregate with labile lyophilic properties and hydration energies. This implies properties of secondness, leading directly to properties of reactive dualism rather than of neutral monism (or of psycho-physical parallel-ism). Hence, the actually experienced dualistic nature of all living organisms depends on the lability of protoplasm, as it exists in reactive heterogeneous physicochemical systems. These do not represent degraded forms of living matter such as inert states of protoplasm, which have lost the properties of irritability or responsiveness. On the contrary, responsive intracellular proto-plasm is essentially dualistic since it is capable of alternating its physicochemical states between limiting states of order or disorder. In this way, it behaves as a dielectric 'valve' connecting organism and environment. Thus, the nerve endings of receptor sensory organs can transmit lyophilic energy by means of oscillations of the intracellular protoplasmic structures. This can be understood only on the basis of reactive dualism rather than as an example of *neutral monism* or of 'preestablished harmony', as in *Leibniz'* doctrine of 'sufficient reason' (chapter 5).

Bifurcation and Unification of Mind and Matter

Descartes' method, as shown by many authors, leads to a bifurcation of nature into realms of mind and matter, of protoplasm and inert matter, and of subject and object in all realms of nature. This bifurcation, however useful, in the objective study of the external physical or non-biological universe, runs into immediate difficulties once it is attempted to reduce the living *phyla* of biology to the dimensions of non-living or inert substance.

The Inscrutable Nature of Reality

All human knowledge of the ultimate reality of living and inanimate nature is derived from sense data received by billions of nerve endings in the peripheral sense organs. These data are then observed by the adult human being as 'perceptions', 'ideas' and 'phenomena', based on faculties of understanding that require empirical experience of all kinds. Hence, the organization of any body of scientific knowledge or phenomena generally passes through a series of approximate descriptive steps, which can be regarded as pure 'phenomenology', consisting mainly in descriptions of the external world.

Then, according to *Eddington* (1929), a threefold process of knowledge is undergone by all students of science: first, the apprehension of the inscrutable ultimate nature of any aspect of physical reality; second, a theoretical or imaginative depiction of this inscrutable reality which is formed by the human mind, and third, the methods of observational experimental scientific research, which must convey increasingly exact information from the objective world to the scientific observer. *Eddington* refers to the experimental data as 'pointer readings'. The advancement of science, including the applications to physiology, biology, and medicine, depends more and more on the development of exact recording devices, as developed in the basic sciences of physics and chemistry.

The physicist deals with basic concepts expressed in words such as 'force', 'angle', 'length', 'velocity', and so forth, which are capable of exact physical measurement. With the progress of science, such concepts tend to become more exactly measurable, and attain the status of 'physical quantities'. As this occurs, each such quantity tends to lose any metaphysical or subjective quality originally assigned to it. Such a quantity is finally definable in terms of the exact physical measurements used in its measurement. In such a case, the given quantity is said to be 'operational' (*Bridgman,* 1927). Otherwise, the quantity or measurement is 'non-operational' and 'meaningless'. These terms refer to the actual 'pointer readings' observed by the physicist, biologist, or physiologist.

It will be noted that the above threefold nature of any such scientific problem is amenable to discussion in terms of *Peirce*'s 'firstness, secondness, and thirdness'. The quality of 'firstness' implies the real existence of a conceptually organized human mind, with the faculties of perception, understanding, and cognition. 'Thirdness' refers to the application of exact physical methods toward improving the operations of 'secondness', particularly in improving the sensitivity of perception, and the accuracy of cognition and understanding.

Thus, the methods of physical science from the periods of *Descartes* to the present have to a great extent depended on the continued advances of 'secondness'. The fundamental relation of firstness to thirdness remains the same, a dualistic relationship between subject and object. If the fundamental nature of the external reality remains inscrutable, the phenomenal world remains inaccessible to the Cartesian methods of reduction. This is the dilemma posed by any solution in terms of 'neutral monism', in which the physical and psychical realms are mutually independent. Subject and object become mutually accessible on a theory of 'protoplasmic reactivity'. This implies that the acts of perception, understanding, and cognition involve changes of hydration energy or lyophilic energy of protoplasm in the human sense organs and neuromuscular system of the human observer (or in his 'secondness'). When such changes occur in the subject, as in studies of human behavior or anthropology), then 'firstness' also partakes of the quality of 'protoplasmic reactivity'. In the fields of anthropology, culture, human psychology, and behavior, exact pointer readings have usually been considered to be superfluous, and the quality of 'thirdness' based on 'physical quantities' has to a great extent been ignored.

Thus, the general problems of Cartesian dualism depend to a large extent on the function of protoplasmic reactivity, as it depends on the functions of protoplasmic reactivity and hydration energy. When protoplasmic receptor nerve endings can react to affect the properties of firstness and thirdness, problems of Cartesian dualism are no longer conceivable in terms of simple location of particles in space and time. The problem becomes either partly or entirely physiological, and a special subject of physicochemical anthropology.

Parallelism

Within a century or two after the appearance of *Descartes' Discourse on Method*, many subsequent philosophers addressed themselves to the problem of psychophysical dualism, which had been posed. None of these attempts has been fully successful, and some have always been obviously unsatisfactory. Formulations of the problem may take two limiting or extreme forms. First, of the psychic and physical aspects of dualism, one or the other may be given priority. If mind, thought or reason is granted priority, then the physiological processes become subordinate. On the other hand, if the psychic properties are subordinate, the result is to accept a kind of mechanistic materialism, which most philosophers have found unacceptable.

A third approach can be denoted that of 'psychophysical parallelism', which results in the preestablished harmony or 'cosmic optimism' of *Leibnitz*. This doctrine, although possibly acceptable to a foremost mathematician such as *Leibnitz,* has little or no appeal to experimental physiologists or to psychologists.

However, when the entire realm of vertebrate and invertebrate phyla is studied, it is evident that many forms of life appear with widely variable aspects of the dualistic relation between organism and environment (*Bernard,* 1878).

Of *Bernard*'s three forms of life, one is completely inert, and life is not evident *(vie latente).* The second form, represented by *vie oscillante,* includes cold-blooded invertebrates and vertebrates, in which physicochemical and physiological conditions are never completely independent of environmental conditions, but in which high degrees of independence may possibly have been attained. In forms of *vie oscillante,* such as marine invertebrates, the life of the organism depends entirely on external conditions, such as temperature, pressure, pH and salinity, which cannot be controlled by the organism. Therefore, these are conditions of 'firstness', which determine all internal properties of secondness — metabolism, growth rates, behavior, and physicochemical state.

Bernard's third form of life *'vie constante',* is that of warm-blooded vertebrates, such as man and mammals, in which internal physiological conditions are largely independent of external conditions — temperature, pressure, and meteorological conditions. Since the physiological and physicochemical state is one of assumed invariance, the psychic condition is free and independent.

In *Bernard*'s words, 'The stability of the *milieu intérieur* is the primary condition for freedom and independence of existence: the mechanism which allows of this is that which ensures in the *milieu intérieur* the maintenance of all the conditions necessary to the life of elements. From this, we know that there can be no freedom or independence of existence for simple organisms whose constituent parts are in direct contact with the environment, and that this form of life is in fact the exclusive possession of organisms which have attained the highest state of complexity or of organic differentiation.

Firstness and Secondness of Protoplasm

Bernard's fundamental distinctions between the properties of *vie oscillante* and *vie constante* can be formulated as a principle of 'inversion of firstness'.

According to basic studies in paleontology (*Huxley*, 1969), early forms of invertebrates began to appear in the Paleozoic (Ordovician) about 450 million years ago. The transition to vertebrates in the form of fishes, amphibia and reptiles may be dated from the Silurian (400 million years) to the Permean (270 million years). Thus, the origin of vertebrate forms can be regarded as an important, but only a partial, step in the transition from *vie oscillante* to *vie constante*. The final step required the appearance of the earliest mammals and birds, which may be dated from the Cretaceous (about 135 million years).

As has been pointed out, this was the final significant step in the 'inversion of firstness' or the transition from *vie oscillante* to *vie constante*. A comparison of the two fundamental forms may be presented as follows:

	Vie oscillante 600 million years	*Vie constante* 135 million years
Firstness	sea water or other waters	protoplasm in constant *milieu intérieur*
Secondness	geological changes of aqueous ambient	reactivity of protoplasm
Type of dualism	firstness of environment; secondness of protoplasmic organism	secondness of environment; firstness of protoplasm

Thus, the inversion of firstness occurred more than 100 million years ago, concurrently with the development of the mammalian, avian or human kidney, with an osmoregulatory function of controlling the composition of the *milieu intérieur*. This made possible the evolution of an invariant organism with respect to chemical composition and chemical potentials of water and electrolytes. In phylogenetic or ontogenetic development, cells and tissues conform to *Gibbs'* phase rule, with one degree of freedom (*Joseph*, 1973).

In contrast to the well-ordered mammalian organism, which is univariant or invariant, the invertebrate organism is relatively disordered. It is characterized by the same number of degrees of freedom as the *milieur extérieur* or sea water, with variable composition, temperature, and pressure. Thus, the invertebrate protoplasm cannot be characterized as free and independent with respect either to firstness or secondness. The composition and behavior of primitive protoplasm stands in biunivocal correspondence with the composition and physicochemical state of the ambient fluid, or the *milieu extérieur*.

Accordingly, in *vie oscillante*, phylogenetic changes cannot occur independently of geochemical, geophysical, or geological development. Both sets of changes must be completely parallel rather than idependent. On the contrary, phylogenetic changes in mammals and birds may operate according to a principle of dualistic parallelism. Phylogenetic and ontogenetic changes may be completely independent of geological changes, as long as the conditions of constraint permit behavioral adaptations. Thus, 'firstness' and 'secondness' of protoplasm and its behavior may remain independent of geological time. This cannot be true in *'vie oscillante'*, where both firstness and secondness are determined by the properties of a variable *milieu extérieur*.

Unification of Organism and Environment

According to the foregoing principles, it is impossible to conceive of any invertebrate or vertebrate organism as existing independently of its environment. Hence, any conceivable bifurcation of nature into an absolute dualism is vitiated by the nature of protoplasmic reactivity. According to this principle, protoplasm in the invertebrate forms of *vie oscillante* is in direct contact with the *milieu extérieur*. However, certain types of protoplasm, particularly in the sense organs and receptors, are exceptions. Thus, nerve endings in the eye, ear or skin are responsive to visual, auditory or tactile sensations. In these regions, neuroplasm shows the property of irritability, resulting in the transmission of afferent stimuli to various higher regions or ganglia. The transmitted stimuli stand in one-to-one biunivocal correspondence with protoplasmic processes in sense organs, nerves, synapses, and ganglia. Thus, organism and environment are unified by reversible protoplasmic processes, and there is no real dualistic bifurcation in living nature. The fundamental distinction between the lower invertebrates and the higher vertebrates is the differentiation which occurred in the Cretaceous. This has been described as an 'inversion of firstness' between organism and environment. It was made possible by the differentiation of the animal organism into many adaptive kinds of organs, cells, and tissues that permitted freedom and independence of external states, as referred to the *milieu extérieur*.

Chapter 3

Carnot's Principle

The principle attributed to *Sadi Carnot* dates from the publication in 1824 of his important monograph *Reflexions sur la Puissance Motrice du Feu.* This is the only scientific publication of the young French engineer; it is the foundation of what is known as the second law of thermodynamics.

Although *Carnot*'s intention was mainly to establish the laws governing the conversion of heat to mechanical work, careful study has shown that the implications of the second law are of very wide and almost universal applications, including many kinds of chemical, physiological, and biological processes, all of which may be considered to be of physicochemical rather than of a vitalistic nature. This point has never been clearly understood by physiologists, biochemists or biologists of the vitalist or (at present) of the mechanist persuasion, who have been unduly influenced by Cartesian or Newtonian views, which are fundamentally mechanistic rather than thermodynamic organismic (*Joseph,* 1973).

Clausius, writing in the years 1848—1862, modified and generalized many of the results of *Carnot,* rectifying the latter's opinion that heat is of the nature of an indestructible material substance. This notion introduced the present idea that heat or thermal energy is of the nature of kinetic motion of atomic or molecular particles. This idea was incorporated into the kinetic theory of *Maxwell* and *Boltzmann,* and later formed the basis of *Gibbs'* (1901) theory of statistical mechanics and of *Einstein*'s (1905—1908) theory of Brownian movement and statistical mechanics. Thus, the 60 years from 1848 to 1908 witnessed the development of the foundations of a physical theory of cause and chance that related the principles of thermodynamics to mathematical theories of causality, chance and probability (*Born,* 1948). Thus, philosophical problems of the relation of human *values* to physical theories of chance and logic became the subject of an important book by the American philosopher and mathematician, *Peirce* (1955).

The principal publication of *Clausius* appeared in 1850, and bore the title *Über die bewegende Kraft der Wärme.* By the year 1869, *Clausius'* ideas were sufficiently clear to enable him to state the principles of thermodynamics in the form: the energy of the universe is constant; the entropy of the universe approaches a maximum.

This motto states with great generality the first and second laws of thermodynamics. The first half of the motto summarizes the views of *von Helmholtz, Joule,* and *Mayer,* enunciated from 1842 to 1847, and fully verified by nutritionists and other physiologists during the ensuing decades. The entropy principle, as stated by *Clausius,* is now known as *Carnot*'s principle or the principle of *Carnot-Clausius.* It is applicable in a very general sense not only to cosmological, geological, and biophysical problems of a very wide range, but also to laboratory experimentation in physical chemistry, physical biology and, as will be shown to animal and human behavior (*Joseph,* 1973). It should be clearly understood that it is the entropy of the *Universe* that approaches a maximum; there is a principle of *negative* entropy (*Boltzmann,* 1905; *Schrodinger,* 1944) that depends on *decreases* of entropy in the biosphere of the earth. This is produced by the synthesis of starches, carbohydrates, and many kinds of polymers of high molecular weight. This depends on processes of photosynthesis in the green leaves of plants. Thus, a large part of the solar energy is retained on the earth in the cells and tissues of plants and animals. This leads to highly evolved, well-ordered systems of low entropy characteristic of living protoplasm. *Carnot*'s principle is thus applicable to the universe as a whole; it does not necessarily apply to the earth, or to any other mass where 'negative entropy' can be retained in cosmic time (chapter 9).

Although at the present time, it is possible to state and apply *Carnot*'s principle in terms of general mathematical formulations involving the theory of Pfaffian differential equations and the properties of line integrals, this was not true until the early decades of the 20th century. Earlier writers on the subject were not always in agreement as to generally valid statements of the principle. Examples of typical 19th century formulations may be noted.

'It is impossible to make a heat engine function with one source of heat' (*Poincaré,* 1903).

'The transformation value of a modification is equal to the diminution that a certain magnitude, connected with all the properties which fix the state of the system, but independent of its motion, undergoes through this modification' (*Duhem,* 1891; *Mouret,* 1896).

It follows from *Duhem*'s statement that: 'Isothermal reversible work in an invariant system is zero' (*Joseph,* 1973).

This also follows from the well-known formula for the maximal efficiency of a heat engine operating between an upper absolute temperature T_2 and a lower absolute temperature T_1:

$$\text{Efficiency} = \frac{T_2 - T_1}{T_2}.$$

Thus, in an isothermal system $(T_2 - T_1)$ and the maximal work become zero (*Carnot,* 1824; *Poincaré,* 1903; *Duhem,* 1891).

A related statement of *Carnot*'s principle has been obtained by *Carathe-odory* (1909) by the use of line integrals for the various thermodynamic functions. In isothermal reversible processes, or in invariant biological systems (homeostasis), the value of any such integral taken over a closed cycle vanishes, with a limiting value of zero. Then for the system as a whole, the principle may be stated: 'there are inaccessible states in the neighborhood of any given state'. *Carnot*'s principle can then be applied to the stability of complex coherent systems, which maintain isothermal invariance, as restricted open systems that may contain metabolizing cells. All cyclic processes may be expressed as line integrals with null values in the limit.

Parmenides and Carnot

In the ancient world, the scientific principle of *causality* or *cause and effect* would have been identified with the principle of immutability of the universe in time. In the search for the causes of phenomena, one invariant guiding principle is that of the persistent identity of the existence of objects in time; the sphere of Parmenides: imperishable and without change.

The Parmenidean doctrine has been shown to resemble or to be analogous with *Laplace*'s conception in many ways (*Meyerson*, 1962). However, the resemblance is quite superficial. The ancient Greek principle of the great Eleatic was one of permanent immutability of an unchanging perfect sphere, in which all internal causal relations were fixed by immutable laws. As a principle of conservation, this is quite analogous to the modern doctrines of the conservation of both matter and energy. The doctrine is a perfect example of the principle that causality or cause-effect relations disappear in a physical system that is completely governed by law. Then causes and effects tend to become identical (chapter 6).

But the nebular hypothesis of *Laplace* (18th century) is incompatible with the idea of the solar system as a conservative system. It is an evolving system, which continually transforms energy from a heat source, the sun at a high temperature T_2, to bodies in other parts of the universe at a low temperature T_1, which in the limit approaches absolute zero. Thus, the solar system, like other parts of the universe, evolves in accordance with *Carnot*'s principle. It is not in thermal equilibrium within itself or with the rest of the universe. Thus, not only the solar system itself evolves with respect to cause-effect relations, but all laws that depend on energy and entropy must be in continual states of evolution. To *Peirce* (1955), we owe the concept of laws that are not immutable, but that depend on the physicochemical and thermodynamic states of an evolving universe. On a cosmological scale, this process may be considered to be observable over periods of geological epochs, involving geology, geophysics and geochemistry. Thus, the cosmic environment and the related biophysical properties must be considered to remain in a slow constant state of evolution, subject to the laws of thermodynamics. In the long run, this must affect the edaphic and biotic conditions that determine the 'fitness of the environment'. Thus, not only physicochemical but also biological laws are in continuous long-term processes of evolution. The modern concepts of causality must be subject to revision, as compared with the immutable principles of identity of causes and effects, as understood in the ancient world by the Greek philosophers. Not only human morphology but also human and animal behavior must evolve according to the principles of chance and logic.

These would be subject to the general conditions of Laplacean evolution of the earth and solar system. The actual laws of hydrodynamic flow would be far more in accordance with the immutable uniqueness of living cells and tissues (*Peirce*, 1892).

Two main classes of intracellular macromolecules have been generally recognized — nuclear or cytoplasmic. These are physically separable and microscopically heterogeneous. They are identifiable by various methods of optical and X-ray spectroscopy, and by the methods of electron microscopy. Theoretical and experimental studies have shown that the molecular kinetic units of both cytoplasm and nucleus are extremely high, with molecular weights of the order of several millions. Thus, the molecular weights of intracellular macromolecules are of higher orders of magnitude than those of such typical soluble extracellular proteins as the serum albumins or globulins, about 70,000—150,000, or of egg albumin, about 40,000 g/mole.

Preparations of these proteins never show the actual properties of living systems, such as irritability, contractility, or reproduction. With few exceptions (those of the filtrable viruses), these properties are confined to intracellular protoplasmic structures composed of heterogeneous colloidal systems of macromolecules, water, and mixtures of physiological ions. These properties, accordingly, cannot be duplicated in the phenomena of 'membrane equilibrium' or 'membrane potentials', as studied with *in vitro* preparations according to the methods of the '*Donnan* equilibrium' (*Donnan*, 1911). The reason for this is that the traditional models of 'membrane equilibrium' apply only to homogeneous solutions with the property of perfect mixing.

Physicochemical systems that are homogeneous, and therefore perfectly mixed, show the property of being relatively unstructured and of high entropy. In heterogeneous systems of the same components, there is little or no mixing and the entropy may be very low. Such properties depend mainly on varying conditions of constraint.

Thus, according to the principles of *Heraclitus,* physical conditions in the universe must involve principles of chance as well as of universal law. In the modern view, the laws of nature, when operative, eliminate chance and causality.

However, when there is absolute freedom in any region of the universe, there is no principle of law, and physical events are entirely random and free of constraints. Normally, in most of the macroscopic physical systems by which we are everywhere surrounded, both kinds of factors are operative.

At all times conditions in the biosphere depend on principles of statistical probability or chance, as well as on immutable principles of cosmology and thermodynamics. The exact extent to which they are subject to chance has been the subject of an interesting written dialogue between two great physicists — *Albert Einstein* and *Max Born* (the *Born-Einstein* letters, 1950). In this exchange, *Einstein* supported the view that physical laws depend on absolute causal necessity, whereas *Born* believed much more firmly in the principles of statistical probability and chance. Historically, *Einstein*'s beliefs would tend to conform to those of the great rationalists of ancient and modern times.

On the other hand, *Born*'s arguments rely more strongly on 19th and 20th century ideas of mathematical or statistical laws of probability. Since the time of *Boltzmann* and *Gibbs,* and of *Einstein*'s own work in statistical mechanics, this has been the prevailing view among physicists. The idea of absolute physical law, however, has found strong support in the latest letter of *Einstein* (1950).

Thermodynamic Functions

Let us assume that a quantity of heat, q calories, is added to a physicochemical system at the constant absolute temperature, T. In the process there is an expansion of the system amounting to ΔV; this increase of volume may be expressed, for example, in liters. Suppose that the pressure, P, is held constant at 1 atmosphere. Then the work of expansion is $P\Delta V$; this amounts to 22.4 liter atmospheres/mole for the assumed process. Then:

$P\Delta V = RT = 22.4$ liter atmospheres at 0 °C.

R is the gas constant; its value is $P\Delta V/T$. This amounts to 22.4/273 = 0.08205 liter atmospheres or 1.987 cal/mole/degree. Thus, the addition of q calories to a gas results in an increase of energy, ΔE, where:

$\Delta E = q - P\Delta V,$

or

$\Delta E = q - w,$

where the work of expansion at constant pressure is expressed as w. Here, neither q or w are functions of state. The true state functions are P, V and T, where each function depends on the other two. Then, at constant temperature:

$P = f (T, V),$
$V = f (T, P).$

For an isothermal gas expansion,

$PV = f (T),$

or

$PV = $ constant.

Therefore, when the gas is expanded by an infinitesimal increase of volume, dV, there is an infinitesimal increase of energy, dE. Then:

$dE = dq - P\, dV.$

In the limit, when the process is isothermal and reversible, dE and P dV are functions of state rather than functions of the path. Therefore,

$dE = T\, dS - P\, dV,$

where S is the molal entropy, a state function, which is independent of the path. Then when E, S, and V are all functions of thermodynamic state rather than of process:

$$\Delta S = \frac{q}{T},$$

where q is the value of the heat increment in an isothermal reversible process, and T is the absolute temperature. The following thermodynamic functions are now defined; each is a function of state rather than of path or process:

$H = E + PV$ (H is the enthalpy),
$A = E - TS$ (A is the work function),
$G = E - TS + PV,$
$\quad = A + PV$ (G is the molal free energy).

Each of the five functions is a true function of state. They are related in the following way:

$dE = T\, dS - P\, dV$ or $E = f (S, V),$
$dH = T\, dS + V\, dP$ or $H = f (S, P),$
$dA = - S\, dT - P\, dV$ or $A = f (T, V),$
$dG = - S\, dT + V\, dP$ or $G = f (T, P).$

Thus, arranged in pairs as above, the four independent variables or *arguments* (E, V, T, and P) yield four related functions (E, H, A, G). The four resulting equations are fundamental and equivalent. Thus, a relation between A, T, and V is equivalent to one between G, T, and P, or to one between H, S, and P. From any one fundamental equation, all the values of the functions E, H, A, and G may be derived. This yields a complete thermodynamic description of the system, as related to any of the four pairs of independent variables. When the quantity of heat, dq calories, is added to a physicochemical system, it can be related to the infinitesimals dE and P dV. Thus:

$$dq = dE - P \, dV,$$

where E, P, and V are defined as in the foregoing. P and V may be taken as independent variables. E, P, and V are functions of thermodynamic state, and therefore form perfect differentials. The infinitesimal dq depends on path or process, and is a state function only in the limit when these are isothermal and reversible. The following integral may be formed as a function of P and V:

$$\int (X \, dV + Y \, dP).$$

When this is extended over a closed path, C, it represents the heat absorbed between an initial state 1 and a final state 2. For a true state function, a line integral becomes zero for a cyclic process in which states 1 and 2 are constant and identical. Then the value of the following integral is found over a closed path to attain a null value when state 1 is exactly the same as state 2. Thus,

$$\int \frac{X \, dV + Y \, dP}{T} = 0$$

(*Born*, 1948; *Caratheodory*, 1909), where T is the absolute temperature. The infinitesimal change of entropy is defined as dS. It can be represented as:

$$dS = \frac{dq}{T} \text{ or } dq = T \, dS,$$

where S is the molal entropy, a state function, and dS is a perfect differential. In any isothermal reversible process:

$$T \Delta S = q = 0.$$

The entropy change, calculated as a line integral for any reversible cyclic process is zero. This is true of the other functions: ΔH, ΔE, ΔA, and ΔG. All can be expressed as reversible cyclic processes, which attain null values in an invariant system. Thus, in the resting state, a biological system represents an invariant heterogeneous continuum rather than an infinite number of cycles. Such a system is conservative, reversible, and invariant. Its state is governed by *Carnot*'s principle and by *Gibbs*' 'equilibrium of heterogeneous substances'.

Maintaining invariant thermodynamic state, it also maintains constant metabolic rates and energies (*Joseph*, 1973). Thus, the fundamental laws of the system are determined by *Carnot*'s principle, rather than by mechanistic processes that are dependent on simple location of material particles.

Accessible States

'There are inaccessible states in the neighborhood of any given state' (*Caratheodory*, 1909; *Born*, 1948). This statement can be accepted as a formulation of *Carnot*'s principle, applicable to the homeostasis of the mammalian or human organism. The normal resting states of standard chemical morphology and basal metabolism may then be regarded as the most accessible states (*Joseph*, 1973). Neighboring states may then represent normal behavioral states of modified physiological activity, as in the absorption of food or digestion. These are 'neighboring accessible states'. Pathological or abnormal physiological states are normally inaccessible, but may represent the limiting boundaries of accessibility. Applying *Carnot*'s principle, as developed in *Gibbs*' 'equilibrium of heterogeneous substances', we may define the condition of homeostasis or maximal accessibility by the following conditions, applicable to water and electrolyte balance. In any heterogeneous system, in which water is distributed among p phases, the most accessible state is characterized by the following conditions for water balance, *Gibbs*' equation 77 (*Gibbs*, 1875, 1928):

$$\mu_{H_2O}{}' = \mu_{H_2O}{}'' \cdots = \mu_{H_2O}{}^p, \tag{1}$$

where $\mu_{H_2O}{}'$ denotes the invariant chemical potential of water.

The p phases are denoted by the p superscripts. Thus, in any such system, there are $(p-1)$ equations of water balance among p chemical potentials. Similarly, there are $(p-1)$ equations of electrolyte balance in a system that contains four different electrolytes ($NaCl$, KCl, $CaCl_2$, $MgCl_2$) in a state of reversible balance (*Joseph*, 1971a, b; 1973). Hence,

$$\mu_{AB}{}' = \mu_{AB}{}'' \cdots = \mu_{AB}{}^p,$$
$$\mu_{AB_2}{}' = \mu_{AB_2}{}'' \cdots = \mu_{AB_2}{}^p. \tag{2}$$

In mammalian cells and tissues, including blood plasma and other fluids of the *milieu intérieur*, two classes of electrolytes are present, binary ($NaCl$, KCl) and ternary ($CaCl_2$, $MgCl_2$). The chemical potential of either class can be expressed as a sum of *ion potentials*. Thus:

$$\mu_{AB} = \mu_A + \mu_B \text{ (in any phase)},$$
$$\mu_{AB_2} = \mu_A + 2\,\mu_B \text{ (in any phase)},$$

where A refers to a cation (Na, K, Ca, or Mg), and B refers to the anion (Cl). It follows from these identities that:

$$\Delta\mu_{Na} = \Delta\mu_K = \frac{1}{2}\,\Delta\mu_{Ca} = \frac{1}{2}\,\Delta\mu_{Mg} = -\,\Delta\mu_{Cl} = \delta, \tag{3}$$

where δ is defined as the *equivalent change of chemical potential* of each of the five physiological ions. Thus, there are four relations among the ion potentials in a system of five kinds of ions distributed between any two phases. Each potential is a thermodynamic function. Therefore, each change of potential $\Delta\mu_i$, can be expressed as a line integral extended over any initial and final states. Then:

$$\Delta\mu_i = \int_1^2 d\mu_i.$$

When this integral is taken over a closed cyclic path, states 1 and 2 are identical. Then:

$$\Delta\mu_i = \int_1^2 d\mu_i = 0.$$

Hence, for a system containing five kinds of ions distributed between two phases:

$$\frac{\Delta\mu_i}{z_i} = \int_1^2 \frac{1}{z_i}\, d\mu_i.$$

In an invariant state of maximal stability,

$$\frac{\Delta\mu_i}{z_i} = \int_1^2 \frac{1}{z_i}\, d\mu_i = 0. \tag{4}$$

Thus, according to *Caratheodory*'s method, the most accessible state is expressed by equations 3 and 4. Other conditions of stability refer to electromotive force, E, and the freezing point of water in phase 1 (equations 5 and 6). Thus:

$$FE + \delta = 0. \tag{5}$$

and

$$\mu H_2 O' - \mu H_2 O^\circ = -5.26\,\Delta, \tag{6}$$

where Δ represents the freezing point depression of blood serum in centigrade degrees, and the constant 5.26 refers to the entropy of fusion of ice, expressed as calories/mole/degree. Equation 5 is of the same form as *Gibbs'* equations 687 and 688, where F is the Faraday constant, and E is expressed in volts. The equivalent change of chemical·potential, δ, is then expressed in joules. When the normal resting potential of an intracellular phase is -80 mV as in skeletal muscle:

$$\delta = 96,500 \times 0.080 = -7,720 \text{ J},$$
$$\delta = 1.85 \text{ kcal}.$$

These approach the normal standard values for resting mammalian skeletal muscle. This is the 'most accessible state'. From the water and electrolyte composition of any phase, referred to the state of blood plasma, it is possible to calculate the following functions that have been described in the foregoing: E, the resting potential, μ_{H_2O}, the chemical potential of water in any phase of the heterogeneous system, the ionization constant of any ion in any phase, the standard chemical potentials of the ions, the action potential, muscular work and tension, and a number of dielectric properties of the system. When as in normal mammalian blood, the freezing point depression is -0.58 °C, the calculated value of the chemical potential of water is -3.05 cal referred to the chemical potential of pure water. All the above properties may be regarded as 'colligative', in that they all depend on the state of aggregation and dielectric constant of water in any well-ordered phase (*Joseph*, 1973).

Maximal Work and Tension

The maximal work of skeletal muscle can be estimated (1) by thermodynamic calculations from the water-electrolyte composition, or (2) from the action potential multiplied by the sodium concentration in moles/kg water (*Joseph*, 1973; *Catchpole and Joseph*, 1974). The change of standard chemical potential, $\Delta\mu_{Na}°$, of sodium between skeletal muscle and blood plasma is about 2.8 kcal/mole. This is estimated from the equation:

$$\Delta\mu_{Na} = \Delta\mu_{Na}° + RT \ln \frac{c_{Na}''}{c_{Na}'},$$

where c_{Na}'' is the concentration in muscle, and c_{Na}' is the extracellular concentration, as determined by analysis. The value of $\Delta\mu_{Na}$ (1.85 kcal) corresponds to a resting potential of -80 mV, as shown previously. Then the maximal work of contraction is determined from the dielectric energy, $c_{Na}''\Delta\mu_{Na}°$:

$$c_{Na}''\Delta\mu_{Na}° = 0.028 \times 2.8 \times 10^3 = 78.4 \text{ cal},$$
$$= 330 \text{ J/kg water}.$$

The water content of the adult human arm muscles is about 250 g/kg muscle. This amounts to 82.5 J for the biceps and brachialis (*Hill,* 1944, 1951). *Hill* has estimated the work capacity of skeletal muscle as 9 kg m for the arm, or as 36 kg m/kg water. This converts to 353 J as the work capacity as calculated from $c_{Na}''\Delta\mu_{Na}°$, the dielectric energy. Thus, as a first approximation, maximal work can be equated with the dielectric energy. Similarly, in the high jump, a record of 2.2 m corresponds to a work capacity of about 90 kg m for a man who weighs 70 kg (*Joseph,* 1973; *Catchpole and Joseph,* 1974).

The dielectric energy or work of contraction is related to a change of state of intracellular water. This passes from a contracted state of low configurational entropy, high configurational free energy, and low dielectric constant to a state of high entropy, low free energy, and high dielectric constant. This signifies a change of state of high order (extension) to one of disorder (contraction). In the highly ordered state, the fibers are structured, and water is in a highly structured state of aggregation. On the other hand, contraction breaks the water structure to a state of disorder, with a dielectric constant that approaches 80, as compared to the value of 30 for the stretched (or structured) fiber.

In general, neuromuscular behavior is attended by changes in order and disorder in the neurological structures, and by changes in all the dielectric properties related to electrical potentials.

Maximal isometric tension in frog, mammalian, and human muscle amount to about 3,000 g/cm² of cross-sectional area. This also corresponds to a change of dielectric energy of about 350 J/kg water. There is a thermodynamic relation between free energy, G, tension, t, and length, l, of an elastic fiber such as a myofibril. In differential form, this is:

$$dG = -\ T\ dS - l\ dt.$$

In an infinitesimal process at constant tension, the external work dG is zero, and:

$$T\ dS = -l\ dt,$$

where T and l are constant. Then,

$$T\ dS = -l\ d\ \mu_{Na}°.$$

In isometric contraction, T dS is positive; then $\mu_{Na}°$ decreases by about 2.8 kcal/mole.

Finally, one obtains by integration:

$$t = 8.6\ c_{Na}''\Delta\mu_{Na}°.$$

Isometric tension, like maximal work, is thus a direct measure of dielectric energy. In mammalian muscle, c_{Na}'' is about 0.03 mole/kg water, and $\Delta\mu_{Na}°$ is about 2.8 kcal, or 11,712 J. Then:

$$t = 8.6 \times 0.03 \times 11,172 = 3,022 \text{ g/cm}^2.$$

The calculated tension agrees well with the values observed in mammalian and frog muscle. All human and animal behavior involves rather complex intramuscular changes of state, involving the dielectric and metabolic properties of water. External work is obtained from reserves of dielectric energy available for muscular contraction. Posture in any behavioral state depends on the varying tensions in resting and active states of systems of muscles. These changes are entropic, and involve coordinated changes in the labile states of aggregation and in the dielectric properties of water and electrolytes (*Joseph*, 1973; *Catchpole and Joseph*, 1974).

Chapter 4

Understanding

As a younger contemporary of *Descartes, John Locke* (1632–1704) was well acquainted with the Cartesian system. As a student at Christ Church College, Oxford, he came under the influence of *John Owen,* dean of the College and vice-chancellor of the university. *Owen* owed his position to the influence of *Cromwell* himself; therefore his views were Puritan and of a broadly tolerant nature. However, English political life was troubled by conflicts resulting from the problems of the Restoration and by related problems of a religious and political nature. *Locke* was always actively involved in these questions, and his philosophical thought was always associated with the political, social, and scientific life of the 18th century, which was an age of Reason and Enlightenment, born of the Century of Genius — the age of *Descartes* and *Newton.*

As a late contemporary of *Descartes,* who was active until 1653, *Locke* was a close student of *Descartes'* method, accepting it in some details, but rejecting or modifying it in other ways. Whereas *Descartes* is to be regarded as an extreme rationalist, placing complete reliance on analytical or mathematical deductions from absolutely clear and distinct ideas based on absolutely unchallengeable premises, *Locke* offers an example of English empiricism at its best. The unchallengeable basic presumptions of the empiricist school are *percepts* rather than *concepts.* Thus, they originate in *objects* as they exist in the external world. *Locke*'s views and philosophy are to a great extent based on sensation and perception as related to human experience. His views resemble those of modern phenomenology or existentialism in which physical reality arises mainly from an objective rather than from a subjective point of view. Human understanding is based on experience rather than on instinctive *a priori* judgements, which have been challenged by 20th century students of human behavior, although admitted or not openly challenged by rationalists, such as *Descartes, Leibnitz,* and *Kant.*

The balance between rationalism and empiricism has shifted toward the *a postiori* side of human understanding as the experimental sciences have progressed from the 17th to the 20th century. This depends on the generally unquestioned belief in the verifiable reality of an external world of eternal objects (percepts) that is independent of a subjective world of concepts. It is the ideal of the physical sciences to regard the world as Parmenidean in nature, i.e. to consist of immutable eternal objects, relations, and laws of causality, which are independent of human or animal emotions, reason or values. This would then become independent of human physiology and of the human sense organs, although *Locke* had shown that the latter were indispensable in the acquisition of experimental knowledge.

The development of 20th century psychology, especially in the regions of child behavior and primitive anthropology, has tended to shift the balance toward internal physiological factors of sensation and perception as a necessary *subjective* side of the question of human behavior and understanding. Thus, the belief of the physical sciences in an order of nature which is the basis of all order in the physical world no longer remains unchallenged. In the 20th century, at least since the time of *Einstein*, the results and concepts of physics may no longer be regarded as absolute, as during the period of *Newton* and *Descartes* up to the 20th century, but are referred to a dualistic set of values, which depend on the nature of the human sense organs, measuring instruments, and the neurological conceptual apparatus. These all exist in a world governed by thermodynamic processes of growth, development, and evolutionary change. This is the world of *Carnot* and *Laplace* rather than the immutable universe of eternal objects and laws of *Parmenides, Newton,* and *Descartes.* That is a universe of immutable reason and logic.

The principle of order in such a universe must depend not only on a well-ordered physical universe but also on well ordered laws of structure and behavior in all biological species. None of the internal or external laws and relationships can be regarded as absolutely fixed or immutable in cosmic space and time, except in the limit.

Perhaps fortunately, this limited region of space-time is the one we habitually inhabit in the laboratory sciences and in our day-to-day activities. However, generalized abstract philosophical thought does not limit itself to these regions. Since the ancient Greeks, philosophical thought has always extended itself to cosmic dimensions of space and time, and to all aspects of human thought, consciousness, experience, and behavior. It is an urgent need of 20th century scientific and philosophical thought to base its phenomenology of understanding on anthropology, which includes all the physical, chemical, phylogenetic, and physiological aspects of human morphology and behavior.

During the period of *Locke*'s activities in philosophy, he was engaged in establishing the basis of his empiricism in scientific methodology. This period likewise coincided with his activities in the fields of political and religious thought and in related fields of human behavior. Thus, *Locke*'s philosophy and scientific activities establish him as a key figure in finding bridges between the various physical, political, and social sciences.

Since these activities occurred largely in the latter years of the 17th century, and continued up to the time of his death in 1704, *Locke* may be regarded as a key figure in establishing bridges between early rationalists such as *Descartes,*

Malebranche, and *LaMettrie* and later figures of the enlightenment such as *Rousseau, Diderot,* and *Voltaire.* The latter groups could be extended to include American philosophers such as *Franklin* and *Jefferson.* All were rationalists in relation to the physical sciences and enlightened empiricists in the political realm.

Locke's activities preceded those of *Laplace* and of *Carnot* by a century or more. Like the physical universe of *Descartes,* his world was controlled by immutable mechanistic laws of cause and effect that were fundamentally invariant and conservationist. Since this resembled the closed conservative universe of *Parmenides,* causal relationships tended to remain invariant and non-evolutionary. It was only in the 19th century that, influenced by *Carnot*'s principle and the nebular hypothesis, it was recognized that the solar system, the earth, and the remainder of the universe were subject to laws that were continually evolving, and that the principles of causality were not necessarily permanently fixed. These views as to the nature of the physical universe were greatly reenforced by developments in the biological sciences that occurred in the latter part of the 19th century, mainly under the influence of *Darwin* and *Huxley.*

The Cartesian method had always been weak, especially in biology, physiology, medicine, and psychology. To a large extent, it tended to reduce the conceptual world to cogitation or to contemplation of clear and distinct *ideas* expressing invariant geometrical or logical relationships. These were dualistic in nature, since they involved the independence of subjective concepts and objective percepts.

The weakness of the Cartesian scheme was perceived by *Leibniz* as well as by *Locke.* As an empiricist, *Locke* recognized that scientific knowledge was largely *a postiori* in nature and dependent on intelligent use of the human sense organs, aided by scientific instruments, such as lenses, prisms, telescopes, and microscopes. By means of the human sense organs, physiological sensations were translated into mental perceptions that originated in the physical universe. Sensations become perceptions only through systematic habits of empiricism. Thus, scientific knowledge is basically *a postiori.* It cannot be greatly extended by pure thought or by Cartesian cogitation. *Locke*'s way of thinking was essential in the questions raised by later philosophers of the enlightenment, such as *Hume, Kant,* and *Leibniz,* and also in the humanistic thought of the *Philosophes.* Combined with later developments in physical and biological sciences, a way was now opened to serve as a bridge between ethical and moral values related to human and animal behavior and the immutable or evolving laws of causality that operate in the physical universe. These must be connected by certain properties of mutual 'fitness' or adaptation (*Henderson,* 1908). Thus, reasonable human thought and behavior ultimately depend on the understanding of a permanently evolving universe of eternal objects, which are ultimately physicochemical in nature, but in which causal relations are sometimes immutable, but are generally involved in evolutionary processes on a geological or cosmological time scale. Understanding of this process depends on rational cogitation aided by systematic application of the principles of phenomenological sensation and perception. Understanding of the cosmic process thus requires both Cartesian dualism and Lockean empiricism. This involves the systematic organization of sensation and perception by the scientific faculties of understanding.

Human Knowledge and Understanding

In the following sections, a number, of representative selections and abstracts will be presented as quotations from the works of *Locke,* or in the form of summaries. It will be attempted to present fair summaries of his general philosophical position by reference to one of his important works, *An Essay Concerning Human Understanding* (1690). This is an important major work, which deals in depth with a number of important subjects related to some of the major problems of 17th century rationalism and empiricism.

Among these topics, *Locke* includes such titles as *Why Men Reason so Poorly, Language and its Proper Use, Liberalism in Politics, The Rejection of Innate Ideas and Principles, The Origin of All Our Ideas in Experience,* and *The Association of Ideas.* This is a very small sample of the topics with which *Locke* chooses to deal, but it indicates the general nature of the material dealing with experience and ideas as the source of knowledge and understanding. The following pages will present some of these topics in the form of brief outlines. Reference to antecedent philosophical views of some of *Locke*'s predecessors and successors will be found in the preceding pages of this chapter.

Why Men Reason so Poorly

Among various common sources of error in applying the faculties of reason, *Locke* enumerated three 'miscarriages' of which men are guilty in reference to their reason which prevent the proper function of these faculties. These 'miscarriages' are found to be quite frequently observed in all men.

(1) The first fault is found in that considerable group who do not reason at all, but who habitually imitate the thought processes of others.

(2) The second common fault is that of putting passion and other common human emotions in place of reason. Such persons 'neither use their own nor hearken to other people's reason any further than it suits their human interest or party'.

(3) The third sort sincerely attempt to follow reason, but lack a 'large,

sound, round about sense ... have not a full view of all that relates to the question'. In short, such people lack the fully rounded views that are the basis for judgements and opinions in difficult questions. Accordingly, they are lacking in experience and keen insights.

According to *Locke*, 'We are all short-sighted, and very often see but one side of a matter; our views are not extended to all that has a connexion with it. From this defect, I think no man is free ... it is no wonder we conclude not right from our practical views.'

In this connection, *Locke* advises frequent consultation with other truth-seekers with varying types of background and experience, so that one is not limited to one type of consultant, one type of book, one type of argument or opinion, or to one type of reasoning or judgement. Sound reasoning then must be based on very wide experience, both of any given reasoner, but also attained at second hand by consultation with friendly or sympathetic advisers. Errors of reason or judgement may then be readily corrected and are less subject to the common types of 'miscarriage'.

The Nature of Language

Man was designed by God to be a sociable creature naturally inclined to communication with his fellows, and also required by vital necessities to do so. For this purpose, not only the organs of speech — mouth, tongue, vocal cords, windpipe and lungs — were requirements. The production of articulate sounds is therefore a natural physiological function which is well ordered, purposeful, and conducive to the development of human reason and understanding. By the use of language, human beings are enabled to communicate ideas and experience, and to develop rational forms of societies and social relations.

Locke was fully aware of the distinction between universals and particulars in the use, for example, of proper nouns and generalized common nouns. This distinction has generally been made in all modern languages that are in common use. Questions as to the absolute reality of universals as distinguished from particulars as objects of thought were topics of debate among nominalists and realists of medieval philosophical and theological circles. It is not surprising, therefore, that *Locke* was familiar with the linguistic aspects of philosophical problems.

Liberalism in Politics

Locke begins this topic by discussing the function of government in main-taining political freedom; this involves consideration of the rights of each individual with respect to property rights and civil liberties. This was later expressed in the American Declaration of Independence as the right of each individual to 'life, liberty, and the pursuit of happiness'. *Locke* arrives at a rational understanding of political power in this way: 'To understand political power aright, and derive it from the original, we must consider what state all men are naturally in, and that this is a state of perfect freedom to order their actions and disposal of their possessions and persons as they think fit, without asking leave or depending upon the will of any other men.' These principles of free government are characteristic of the more liberal constitutional monarchies and of the United States of America, as expressed in the Constitution and Bill of Rights.

Ultimately, *Locke* appears to identify this ideal state of freedom with an imaginary 'state of nature', in which the basic physiological, psychological and social needs are readily satisfied. This would recognize the territorial rights of each individual and of the entire community. The right to a given territory free of the aggressive behavior of neighboring individuals seems to be recognized also by many mammalian species as well as by communities of human beings. Therefore, animal societies or communities (biocoenoses) appear generally to recognize individual rights in much the same way as do free human societies (*Wheeler*, 1928; *Bourlière*, 1953; *Lorenz*, 1970, 1972).

Innate Ideas and Principles

At all times, according to *Locke*, there seem to have been groups of men, including philosophers, who have held to the opinion that human beings enter the world at birth, equipped with sets of innate or congenital ideas, which are independent of their later experience. *Locke* argues strongly and convincingly against this opinion, supporting the opposite opinion that nature offers no congenital supply of ideas that are independent of education and nurture during the years of infancy and early education.

The beliefs urged by *Locke* were accepted by all philosophers of the empiricist school, especially in England. Empiricists generally reject innate ideas and principles as a basis of knowledge and belief. These ideas are acquired rather than inherited. Since the time of *Lamarck*, competent biologists have generally rejected the principle of the inheritance of acquired characteristics as applied to vertebrate or mammalian biology in general. The Lamarckian school, like its counterparts in philosophy, appear to have been completely discredited since the early 19th century. For recent 20th century opinion on the questions raised by empiricists since *Locke*, and rationalists since *Descartes*, it is necessary to consult the recent observations by *Piaget* (1970), as outlined in chapter 10 (Growth of the Mind).

Locke, like all other philosophers of both rationalist and empiricist beliefs, accepts the necessary coexistence of mind and body. In relation to the thesis of chapters 1—9 of the present volume, thought and behavior, are coexistent with the principles of human anatomy, physiology, and biochemistry. These special sciences may be regarded as branches of the main subject described by the title *Structural and Chemical Anthropology.* Structural anthropology, including chemical morphology, is the permanent substructure of all human behavior. These are fundamentally secondary rather than primary properties. They evolve with the development of human culture and societies.

Thus, thought and behavior develop according to Darwinian rather than Lamarckian laws and principles. This fact obliges us to reject, with *Locke,* the existence of innate or congenital ideas. Like *Locke,* we are likewise compelled to reject the existence of 'clear and distinct ideas' as the basis of a rationalized science in any field other than pure mathematics. According to empiricist principles, even such sciences as algebra and geometry originated and developed in relation to human experience rather than on a basis of *a priori* rationalism.

Thus, the attempts by logicians to derive mathematics from the logic of classes and relations have generally been rejected by many authorities on scientific philosophy (*Poincaré,* 1946; *Mach,* 1942). The works of *Frege and Cantor* and others of the logical school have generally resulted in insoluble paradoxes. The general reason for the termination of the efforts of the rational school was finally advanced by *Godel* in 1932, himself a product of the school founded by *Frege and Cantor.* One important development of the line of thought initiated by *Cantor* was the theory of sets and aggregates. This line of thought has led to new lines of mathematical formulation, resulting in important types of graphical representation of physicochemical systems of the kind studied in general physiology (*Henderson,* 1928; *Joseph,* 1971a, b; 1973). These take the form of Cartesian and d'Ocagne nomograms. These depend on general principles of analytical geometry, but they also depend on empirically derived physicochemical data. They can hardly be regarded as attempts to reduce the physiological sciences to a rationalist basis. They require the application of Lockean as well as Cartesian principles, and are not to be confused with other aspects of the Cantorian doctrines, such as the theory of transfinite numbers (*Joseph,* 1973).

The Idea of Number

The simplest idea of number that can be entertained by the human mind is unity or one. Each thing or subject is expressed by this number, into which any whole number whatever can be resolved. Thus, the number one is the class of all units; one man, one dog, one egg, one loaf of bread or one tree. It is the class of all invariant simple units. Similarly, the number of four is the class of all quartets or groups of related objects of the same kind. A string quartet; the seasons in a year; the points of the compass; the players in a game of bridge. There is a one to one correspondence between members of two different quartets. Thus, in a game of bridge, one may refer to the various players as North, South, East, and West. They might as readily be enumerated as Spring, Summer, Autumn, and Winter.

This simple mode of expression enables us to resolve the simplest ideas of mathematical thought into ordinary grammatical language. It is also the method of obtaining any series of numbers by the simple addition of one unit. Thus, any quartet is related to the corresponding trio by the addition of one unit of the same kind.

By simple self-evident reasoning of this kind, *Locke* adduced the principle of *Simple Modes of the Idea of Number*. Extension of the idea would yield the self-evident result that an octet is the sum of two quartets. Such results apply to the usual sort of identical invariant relations found in elementary arithmetic, as studied by children in the first years of grammar school.

According to *Locke*, such thinking is not innate. One learns how to count, to measure and to weigh by empirical procedures. Thus, one counts the number of grams in a pound, the number of meters in a mile, the number of inches in a meter, by simple invariant ratios of fundamantal units. Quantitative science of any kind is based on these well accepted standard procedures. The origin of such procedures seems to be of a practical or economic nature, such as in measuring or surveying land (with respect to areas or distances). According to *Poincaré* (1946), the kind of mathematics used in science requires mainly this practical foundation rather than a study of logical origins, as attempted by *Frege* and *Russell*. Experience has shown that such a rationalist approach usually leads to insoluble paradoxes (*Godel*, 1967).

In his *Introduction to Mathematics, Whitehead* (1911) describes the essential foundations of mathematics in much the same way as that employed by *Locke* about two centuries earlier. Thus, in this work he is in essential agreement with the traditional empirical approach. However, at about the same time, *Whitehead and Russell* published the standard work *Principia Mathematica*, in which a foundation for the principles of mathematics was sought in logic.

A new basis was sought in symbolic methods. The results, although very impressive, contained some paradoxical material, the solution of which required further efforts. For about 30 or 40 years, various paradoxes were found in the earlier work of *Frege, Richard, Burali-Forti, Zermelo* and many others. In general, these seem to involve fundamental linguistic difficulties. Perhaps they are inherent in attempts to find an absolutely rational basis for pure mathematics. Possibly they are analogous to the ancient paradoxes of *Zeno*. These are logically flawless, but they defy empirical common sense, and are therefore mathematically unsound. In general, one may accept unequivocally *Locke*'s views as to the nature of numbers and mathematics.

The Nature of Ideas

The ideas of any man are best known to himself alone by what we may call 'introspection'. Such introspective ideas can be but roughly or crudely communicated to others by articulate spoken language or by written symbols.

By the 'nature of ideas', *Locke* means their causes and manner of production in the mind. Since *Locke* denies the existence of innate ideas, the origin of all ideas in the human mind is *a postiori* rather than *a priori.* This applies to such general ideas as numbers, quantity and measureable magnitudes, which arise by one-to-one correspondences between articulate and written words and what is learned about classes of numerical aggregates, such as trios, quartets, quintets, sextets and octets. Thus, the concept of number in the mind is associated with processes of counting. This begins with the child's discovery of his five fingers on each hand and that the total number is ten. Finally, this leads to the invention of mechanical computers of many kinds, whose operations correspond to those of the mind (*Wiener,* 1948).

Thus, the notion of 'idea' is associated with the origin of ideas in the mind. This process begins in sensation as localized nerve endings in the eye, ear, skin, olfactory organs, or those of taste, and are finally perceived by a process of *understanding,* which depends on organized experience. Comprehended ideas of this kind are then communicated from one person to another through articulate or written language, in such terms as sweet, bitter, loud, soft, and so forth. In the growth of the human mind, communication of ideas begins in childhood at an age which depends on nurture and instruction rather than on innate aptitudes.

Chapter 5

Skepticism

At the root of all scientific investigations, there are certain fundamental doubts as to the validity of any scientific theory, presumably based on the availability of exact quantitative measurements. This has been explained by *Eddington* in his *The Nature of the Physical World* (1929). In chapter 12, entitled *Pointer Readings, Eddingston*'s explanations proceeds in the following way: 'As the exact sciences, physics and chemistry, have come to depend more and more on the use of accurate measuring devices, their progress depends on the triple correspondence: (a) the image formed in the human mind but which is not in the external world; (b) an inscrutable counterpart in the external world; (c) a set of pointer readings determined by exact science and related to other sets of readings.'

The principal quantities with which the physicist deals are expressed by concepts such as length, angle, mass, and so forth. In the early stages of any physical science, some of these concepts are metaphysical or 'non-operational' in nature. In the course of time, the definitions become more and more exact and uniform; the units become better standardized, conforming to actually observable physical magnitudes. According to *Bridgman* (1927), all significant definitions and measurements must be 'operational', and must be free of undefinable and immeasurable concepts or steps. When this limit is attained, the sets of pointer readings in *c* may be brought into fairly exact agreement; this is necessary to bring the corresponding images or ideas in the human mind into more approximate agreement. Finally, as the sets of pointer readings and mental images are brought into agreement, concepts and percepts can be thought to correspond with reasonable accuracy. The final step in scientific thought is that of bringing concepts into exact agreement with the hitherto inscrutable counterpart that is thought to exist in the external world.

This process corresponds with *Locke*'s empiricist theory of human knowledge, based on the origin of human ideas in the external world. In modern physics and chemistry, the sensations of the eye and ear are greatly amplified by the systems of pointer readings obtained by the use of lenses, prisms, mirrors, and so forth, as well as by vacuum tubes, amplifiers, and other accurate devices.

As these are improved, concepts, percepts, and understanding are brought into more perfect harmony. In the limit, *skepticism* tends to vanish.

David Hume (1711–1776)

Of the great English empiricists of the 18th century, *Hume* ranks as a preeminent figure of the enlightenment, along with *George Berkeley* as a representative of subjective idealism. *Locke, Hume,* and *Berkeley* were prominent in the political, religious, social, and moral problems of their age. These were regarded as involving questions of human knowledge, understanding, and values. Five principal philosophical works are attributed to *Hume:* (1) *A Treatise of Human Nature* (1739–1740); (2) *An Inquiry Concerning Human Understanding* (1748); (3) *An Enquiry Concerning the Principles of Morals* (1754); (4) *On the Standard of Taste* (1757), and (5) *The Natural History of Religion* (1757).

The birth of *Hume* (1711) is dated 7 years later than the death of *Locke.* Covering a period of about 20 years between 1739 and 1757, many of the problems dealt with by *Hume* were of a similar nature to those which occupied *Locke* during the second half of the 17th century. However, the backgrounds of the two philosophers differed in several respects. *Hume,* in comparison with *Locke,* is said to have been an indifferent student of the natural sciences and of mathematics. Both philosophers were ardent students of *Descartes'* method, but as empiricists, were not his followers. *Locke* believed much more strongly in the efficacy of the physical sciences, based on the reality of abstract principles. As a philosopher, he is to be classed with medieval realists such as *Roger Bacon* and *Duns Scotus.*

On the other hand, *Hume* is much more clearly allied with medieval nominalists, such as *Peter Abelard* and *William of Occam,* and with skeptical thinkers of the later renaissance, such as *Montaigne.* The realist position in medieval life accepted a direct correspondence between universals in nature and human thought based on direct intuition of perception. Thus, abstract universal ideas were not manifested through direct perception. In *Plato*'s image, they were perceived indirectly — as shadows in a cave. Thus, in *Eddington*'s formulation, they appeared in the human mind as inscrutable realities, manifested only as intermediate pointer readings.

To minds such as *Abelard, Occam,* and *Descartes,* the reality of such intangibles as the immutable truths of religion, morals, and human institutions was questioned. Thus, nominalists such as *Abelard* and *Occam* accepted only the existence of particular, tangible objects. Fundamentally, they would have agreed that the mind of the subject is different in nature from the nature of the tangible external object. This view can lead to profound skepticism of the kind felt by *Hume,* as a result of his studies of human nature.

George Berkeley (1685–1753)

George Berkeley, DD, Bishop of Cloyne, was well known, to various kinds of readers during the 18th and 19th centuries, and has continued to maintain an important place in philosophy up to the present time. Despite an air of levity somewhat surprising in a bishop, he continues to attract serious readers. At first sight, some of his metaphysical principles seem rather paradoxical, but close scrutiny shows him to have disclosed some hitherto unrevealed aspects of philosophical thought.

For example, he affirms the existence of Platonic ideas and universals, while denying the existence of matter, our inability to perceive spatial distances and form, and other kinds of spatial and temporal relations. He has always been known for a special kind of adroitness in presenting his ideas, but these have not always been acceptable to many readers. His denial of the general theory of ideas, knowledge and understanding that we owe to *Locke* and *Hume* commits him to a realist rather than to a nominalist position in philosophy. As becomes a bishop, this allies him with medieval theologians of the Platonic tradition, *Duns Scotus,* for example, rather than with nominalists such as *Abelard, Occam,* and *Hume.* This inclines them towards skepticism in their beliefs as related to the reality of abstract universals in other than a formal or linguistic sense.

According to *Whitehead* (1925), the problem of simple location of any entity or object is at the core of *Berkeley*'s philosophy, which is characteristic of subjective idealism. This separates him from other thinkers of the period, such as *Locke* and *Hume,* and further isolates him from inheritors of their tradition, such as *Leibniz* and *Kant,* who owe little or nothing to subjective idealism. This, in effect, criticizes the traditional notion of simple location (an idea accepted by *Descartes* and *Locke*). *Berkeley* raises the question of the realization of things in the world of nature.

In certain sections of his *Principles of Human Knowledge, Berkeley* gives answers to the following questions:

(1) 'But, say you, surely there is nothing easier for me to imagine trees, for instance, in a park, or books existing in a closet, and nobody by to perceive them. I answer, you may say there is no difficulty in it; but what is all this, I beseech you, more than forming in your mind certain ideas, which you call books and trees, and at the same time omitting to frame the idea of any one that may perceive them?

'When we do our utmost to conceive the existence of external bodies, we are all the while only contemplating our own ideas. But the mind, *taking no notice of itself,* is deluded to think it can and does conceive bodies existing unthought of or without the mind, though at the same time thay are apprehended or exist in itself ...

'It is very obvious upon the least inquiry into our thoughts, to know whether it is possible for us to understand what is meant by the absolute existence of sensible *objects in themselves,* or *without the mind.* To me it is evident that those words mark out either a direct contradiction, or else nothing at all.'

(2) *Whitehead* further quotes a 'remarkable passage' from *Berkeley*'s *Alicphon.*

Euphrenor: Tell me, Alicphon, can you discern the doors, window and battlements of that same castle?

Alicphon: I cannot. At this distance it seems only a small round tower.

Euph.: But I, who have been at it, know that it is no small round tower, but a large building with battlements and turrets, which it seems you do not see.

Alc.: What will you infer from thence?

Euph.: I would infer that the very object which you strictly and properly perceive by sight is not that thing which is several miles distant.

Alc.: Why so?

Euph.: Because a little round object is one thing, and a great square object is another. Is it not so?

Berkeley's clever paradoxes make it clear that he adopts an extreme idealistic interpretation. Mind is the only absolute reality, and the unity of nature exists only in the mind of God. Natural laws are then interpreted as inscrutable and inaccessible to the human sense organs and become comprehensible only as a divine idea. *Locke*'s theory of the empirical nature of ideas, reason, and scientific knowledge seems to disappear, along with the conventional concept of causality. Thus, subjective idealism is compatible with the ideas of the medieval schools of Platonists and theological scholasticism, but do not conform to the main lines of empirical development of the Cartesian method by *Locke, Leibniz,* and *Kant.*

Berkeley's subjective idealism, although incompatible with Cartesian dualism, nevertheless opens paths, unknown to *Berkeley,* which are consonant with organicist and structuralist rather than Cartesian or Kantian thought. These paths depend on non-empirical realist modes of perception. This implies thought processes that are independent of simple location of particular objects in space and time. It also implies the occurrence of all physical or biological processes in a well-ordered purposeful universe, in which laws of nature are not denied, but in which they operate in accordance with the principles of *Laplace* and of *Carnot.* The processes operate under principles of reversibility, as well as under irreversible or evolutionary conditons. On a cosmic scale, the universal processes are inaccessible to observations in any local regions of space-time.

Comprehension of such cosmic processes must involve the principle of subjective idealism *(Berkeley)* rather than that of nominalistic empiricism *(Occam, Locke, Hume).* Further elaboration of the problem would require application of the thought of *Peirce* (1878, 1892), *Whitehead* (1925, 1929),

Bridgman (1927) and *Eddington* (1929). Biological and behavioral aspects would then require reference to the ideas of *Lorenz* (1970, 1972) and of *Merleau Ponty* (1962).

Inductive Inference

Three main types of inference may be represented by affirmative syllogisms of the following types (*Peirce,* 1892):

(a) Analytical or deductive;
(b) Hypothesis;
(c) Inductive.

These types are illustrated by the examples:

Rule (a) all S is M;
Case (b) all M is P;
Result (c) therefore all S is P,

where S stands for subject, P for predicate, and M for the middle term.
As an example:

Rule: all muscles can contract;
Result: M can contract;
Case: therefore M is a muscle.

Inductive inference, instead of obtaining a general rule from two known premises, attempts to infer a given case from a particular result. This is the general procedure in experimental science. As is known by all capable experimenters, the success of any inductive inference depends on a factor of chance or probability. This in turn depends on the sampling procedure. If, as in the above example, the number of samples includes only specimens of contractile muscle, the induction becomes valid. If, however, M includes, in addition to samples of contractile muscle M', samples of elastic rubber bands M'', the validity of the inference depends on the ratio of M' to M''. If M' is a finite number, and M'' is zero, then:

$$P = \frac{M'}{M'} = 1.0.$$

In this case, the probability of the inference is 1.0, which amounts to saying that there is no chance of error. If, however, M' is 50 and M'' is also 50,

$$P = \frac{M'}{M' + M''} = \frac{1}{2}.$$

Then the probability of any given sample being a specimen of muscle is one half. The probability of any induction being valid is given as a ratio of the number of the given kind of samples to the total number. Modern theories of statistical probability depend on mathematical methods developed in the 19th century by the use of the Gaussian curves of probable error. Experimentalists generally express their results in terms of mean values, with a standard error (SE) of plus or minus so many units. Only as SE approaches zero, do the results approach certainty.

In physics, such a result has been obtained from measurements of the wavelength of the monochromatic red line of cadmium. The error is of the order of one part in a billion. The wavelength can be expressed to nine significant figures. Many physical and biological measurements are significant only to one part in ten or one part in a hundred. Errors of this magnitude occur due to the uncertainties of the inductive method.

Hume, it must be pointed out, was a rather indifferent mathematician, and he wrote about a century earlier than the development of modern statistical methods; hence, his distrust of inductive inference was very great. It has been said by many writers that it is not absolutely certain that the sun will rise tomorrow. According to the nebular hypothesis, the origin of the planet Earth may be estimated as occurring about 2 billion years ago. This amounts to about 700 billion days. The lifetime of the earth may be of the order of another 100 billion days. Thus, the possibility of its extinction on any given day might be estimated as of the order of 10^{-9} or 10^{-10}. Thus, we cannot be absolutely certain that there will be a sunrise or sunset on any given day. *Hume*'s extreme skepticism with regard to the certainty of scientific knowledge is based on his general attitude toward the principles of inductive reasoning. In general, this makes him a skeptic in regard to universals, as contrasted with particulars. As noted by *Gilson* (1937), *Hume*'s nominalism and his skepticism are allied with the nominalistic empiricism of *William of Occam.*

Despite *Hume*'s skepticism toward experimental science, practical investigators have paid scant attention to his general criticisms. As a philosopher, *Hume* was mainly interested in political science, morals, and ethics, which are not quantitative inductive sciences. They are based on a profound interest in human nature as such, rather than as statistical norms of human behavior. Statistical curves of behavior would undoubtedly reveal SEs of high magnitude. Reproducibility of such statistical curves would predictably be low. In this field, *Hume*'s skepticism would be amply justified. This is true also of *Berkeley*'s faith in subjective idealism, as contrasted with the validity of concrete observations. The views of both *Hume* and *Berkeley* could be regarded as parts of the general subjectivist attack on Cartesian and Lockean dualism (*Lovejoy,* 1960).

The Attack on Cartesianism

According to *Descartes,* the essential property of matter is extension. This is a geometrical idea, suitable for expression of physical conceptions in a mathematical framework. According to the method, it serves as a clear and distinct idea adaptable to theoretical development as an *a priori* principle, for example, to the science of kinematics, expressed as simple location of material particles in space and time. In Newtonian physics, this idea was developed in the 17th and succeeding centuries to include all of theoretical mechanics, as well as kinematics.

From the Cartesian and Newtonian systems, it is possible to extend these ideas to include most of the essential elements of physical reality. These principles were at the core not only of theoretical mechanics, optics, acoustics, and electromagnetism at least until the end of the 19th century. After the time of *Clausius, Maxwell, Boltzmann,* and *Einstein,* the theory of heat could also be expressed as an aspect of simple location of elementary particles. The entire line of development can be traced to its origin in the 17th century. The outstanding exception in the sciences was physical or chemical thermodynamics, which to a large extent can be developed independently of the principle of simple location of particles in space and time. Thermodynamic state depends not only on the motions of particles, but also on order, disorder, and state of aggregation of any physicochemical system. *Carnot*'s principle dates from a period almost two centuries later than *Descartes*' method.

While serving as the indispensable basis for most of the physical sciences, at least until the middle of the 19th century, Cartesian dualism was by no means adequate for the biological and behavioral sciences. The fundamental reason for this, as pointed out by *Locke* and *Leibniz* among others, was the omission of the sense organs and of human sensations and perceptions. *Descartes*' conception of human understanding was primarily rational rather than empirical. This deficiency in the method aroused skepticism in the minds of *Locke, Hume,* and *Berkeley* during the 18th century, and among post-Kantian philosophers, such as *Schopenhauer* and *Nietzsche.* The reason for this is that *Hume* and *Berkeley* were basically interested in human nature and human values rather than in mathematical abstractions such as kinematics. This was also true of *Schopenhauer* and *Nietzsche,* who introduced into their philosophies concepts such as will, power, purpose and voluntarism.

However, until our own time, there have continued to be many biologists who continue in the attempts to reduce biological reality or questions of human values to problems conceived of as mechanistic positions of elementary particles in space and time. This approach tends to be mechanistic and Cartesian; it tends to underestimate ideas related to organization, 'givenness', and other concepts related to entropy, free energy, and other derivations from *Carnot*'s principle.

Then it would be impossible to account for evolutionary changes of morphology, structure, and behavior simply in mechanistic formulations that date from *Descartes* and *Newton.*

Locke, Hume, and *Berkeley* were much more biologically and anthropologically oriented, and interested in problems of value and behavior. Thus, they provide valuable bridges to 20th century biology and psychology, which have advanced greatly beyond 19th century conceptions (as in *Piaget*'s *Child Psychology* and *Levi-Strauss' Primitive Anthropology*). Advances have also been made in the *Principles of Animal and Human Behavior* (*Lorenz,* 1970, 1972). The concepts of *Emergent Evolution* might also be cited (*Wheeler,* 1928). All of these developments would lend themselves to expression in organicist rather than in mechanistic terms. Thus, the 19th century attempts to replace 'vitalism' by 'mechanism' seem to have had the result of developing a kind of Cartesian neo-vitalism (*Joseph,* 1973). In this connection, it is possible to quote *Sarton* (1952): 'It is impossible to suppress the vitalist point of view. It dodges every blow and appears under a new form.'

The long-lasting survival of vitalism in the guise of mechanism is due, from the foregoing considerations, to the rather amazing survival of dualism in its Cartesian form. A 20th century revival of the attack on simple location in a mechanistic universe would require a corresponding revival in the humanism of *Locke* or in the subjective idealism of *Berkeley (Plato, Duns Scotus, Peirce).* The corresponding struggle between subjectivism and objectivism will, according to this, require fundamental revisions in human value judgements (*Whitehead,* 1925, 1929).

'Secondness of Extension'

In the 20th century, the idea of extension in space, rather than being regarded as a primary property of matter, has tended to be regarded along with all other geometrical properties as of a secondary nature. Thus, if motion is taken as primary, then velocity is taken as the first derivative of a coordinate with respect to time. This applies either to linear or to angular displacements. Acceleration, or force, is then taken as the first derivative either of a linear velocity, one of its components, or of angular velocity. Thus, any force of acceleration can be expressed as a second derivative of a spatial coordinate with respect to time.

From this point of view, spatial extension is secondary, and motion is primary. It follows that the Newtonian conception of absolute space and time is a useful conception rather than an irreducible or immutable natural principle.

If physical reality is conceived of as natural processes or events rather than as secondary manifestations of simple location (according to *Descartes*), then it follows that, contrary to the method, extension of matter in space is *not* a clear and distinct idea. This Cartesian concept must be replaced by a scheme in which the primary processes or events are the *motions* or *energies* of given groups of entities in n-dimensional space. Thus, the fundamental natural realities are *events* or *processes* in non-Euclidean or hyperdimensional space of *n* dimensions (*Whitehead,* 1929).

Applied to natural phenomena in a biological universe, sets and subsets of morphological and metabolic processes cannot be isolated *in any sense of identification* (*Spaulding,* 1919; *Wheeler,* 1928; *Joseph,* 1973). This is the basic idea of the science of emergent evolution, as it must be conceived in the sciences of physical biology or ecology. The idea of *process* is thus antagonistic to that of Cartesian dualism. The latter idea, as has been shown in the preceding section, leads to a kind of neo-vitalism, as a product of mechanistic simple location. This can be avoided by basing the biological conceptual scheme on *Carnot*'s principle rather than on one based on localized mechanisms. *Carnot*'s principle is capable of unifying heterogeneous structures in physicochemical systems into well-ordered morphological entities. This is impossible with mechanistic systems of the neo-vitalist imagination. These rely on the multiplication of non-observable *ad hoc* entities. In so doing, they violate *Occam*'s razor, 'entities are not to be multiplied without necessity'. In addition, they exemplify *Whitehead*'s 'fallacy of misplaced concreteness'. Both these faults are avoided by the use of *Carnot*'s principle and *Gibbs' Equilibrium of Heterogeneous Substances* (*Joseph,* 1971a, b; 1973).

Chapter 6

Causality

'The law of causality, I believe, like much that passes muster among philosophers, is a relic of a bygone age, surviving, like the monarchy, only because it is erroneously supposed to do no harm.'
Bertrand Russell.

The survival of this relic (the law of causality) has continued at least until the second half of the 20th century, and can be predicted to continue probably indefinitely later into the distant future. The belief must have deep reasons in the anthropomorphic and anthropocentric origin of all human thought and behavior. Thus, describing my own behavior, I could say: 'The wooden chair is in the corner, because I placed it there this morning.' This, of course, is a commonplace statement of fact; the statement would be acceptable even to a Bishop *Berkeley,* but it does not survive the critical skepticism required by modern science and phenomenology. These disciplines are now cognizant of the attacks on Cartesian dualism that have recurred in Europe and America since the time of *Locke, Hume,* and *Berkeley.* To understand the survival of causality as a philosophical or scientific principle, it is necessary to consider the nature of the belief at the height of its fashion in the enlightenment, as during the periods of *Locke* and *Kant.*

Kant's Understanding of Causality

The central point of *Kant*'s definition of causality may be summarized as follows: (1) every event has a cause; (2) the cause of any event is a preceding event; (3) these principles are known to us *a priori.*

Point 3, that our knowledge of causality is *a priori,* is of course the opposite of the view of *Locke* that all human knowledge is empirical and *a posteriori.* *Locke*'s position would agree with that derived from studies of child psychology *(Piaget)* and from those of primitive anthropology *(Levi-Strauss).* Accordingly, the common use of cause-effect relations should be related to the structure of behavior *(Merleau Ponty).* In common sense usage, the concept of causality tends to relate to the sciences of anthropology and ethology, rather than to the non-biological sciences of physics, chemistry, meteorology and geology, for example. In the study of the latter sciences, the concept of causality tends to disappear, and to be replaced by natural law. Since the time of *Newton,* this has been the prevailing belief in the physical aciences, where conspicuous departures from law would be regarded to be of the nature of miracles or supernatural phenomena. Thus, the modern scientific mind tends to regard unnatural causality as either anthropological (magic or contrived deception) or as extrasensory or superstitious. Such beliefs are subject to skepticism by serious students of the physical sciences.

As a universal scholar and philosopher on all human subjects and their origins, *Kant* was quite familiar with the Cartesian identification of causality with natural grounds, with the Leibnitzian principle of sufficient reason (chapter 6), and with *Hume*'s conception of the temporal succession of causes and effects. However, *Kant* seems to have neglected or underestimated the principal presupposition of Newtonian and post-Newtonian physics — this is the doctrine that what happens according to a law happens without a cause. In *Kant*'s *Critique of Pure Reason,* he appears to follow the example of the English empiricists, *Locke* and *Hume,* rather than that of *Newton,* who emphasizes law rather than causality. It should be noted that *Locke* and *Hume* were primarily students of reason as related to human nature or to the biological sciences, rather than as related to the inorganic cosmos, as studied by *Newton* and his followers.

It should also be noted that the concept of law tends to displace the concept of causality in the science of thermodynamics, as exemplified in the principles of *Clausius-Carnot* and of *Joule, Helmholtz,* and *Mayer (Joseph,* 1973). Attempts to replace these principles by those of *Descartes* or of *Newton* always seem to result in a form of neo-vitalism in the guise of mechanism. In these forms of pseudo-biological science, the concepts of mechanistic causality are invoked to replace the laws of thermodynamics. Thus, concepts such as 'ion pumps' or 'ion carriers' always seem to be anthropomorphic or anthropocentric in origin. This often is characteristic of causal explanations in biology, which depend on a 'fallacy of misplaced concreteness'. Such fallacies occur when scientists apply their inductive methods to situations which require analytical reasoning from scientific law *(Newton, Carnot-Clausius),* as well as to the more fallible types of synthetic inference (hypothesis or induction).

The Relation of Leibniz to Kant

It is well known that *Leibniz* (1644–1714), during the later years of his life, was in direct communication with *Locke,* and that both he and *Kant* were influenced by *Locke*'s views on the non-existence of innate ideas. Thus, both German philosophers were motivated in their quests for the principles of reason and causality by English empiricism as well as by French rationalism *(Descartes, Bayle, Malebranche)*.

Unfortunately, *Leibniz* was not generally a writer of well-organized systematic texts, written for the enlightenment of the philosophical and scientific elite of his day. Mostly his writings were of the nature of personal correspondence, abstracts, and articles in the Paris *Journal des Savants,* and elsewhere. These, scattered through scientific and philosophical journals in France, Holland, England, and Germany, constitute a formidable output, later compiled by various editors of collected works, published during the 19th and 20th centuries. A considerable mass of *Leibniz'* voluminous output has, since his death, remained in the permanent collections of the Royal Library of Hanover, where he served as philosophical consultant, historian, and in other capacities. A complete edition of the works of *Leibniz,* including all the papers in the Library of Hanover, is said to be in course of publication under the direction of the Akademie der Wissenschaften of Berlin.

To obtain an idea of the scope and versatility of *Leibniz'* activities in the world of science, philosophy, and human affairs, it is sufficient to list a few of his better known activities. He is best known perhaps for his invention (1675) of the infinitesimal calculus, for which he shares credit with *Newton. Leibniz* is also known as the inventor of a calculating machine and other mathematical inventions. In logic, he is regarded as a formulator of the principle of sufficient reason, later to be elaborated by *Schopenhauer* (chapter 7).

In philosophy, he was critical of the views of *Locke* as to the basis of human understanding. *Bayle*'s views relating to the religious issues of the period were also brought under scrutiny, as *Leibniz* formulated his own teleological doctrine of cosmic optimism. This is expressed in his belief that we live in the best of all possible worlds. This belief is related to the other aspects of *Leibniz'* metaphysics, expressed in the monadology and in the doctrines of preestablished harmony and of preformation.

Cartesian views as to the conservation of mechanical force in nature, and as to the nature of matter itself were also criticized by *Leibniz* and revised by him. Finally, in relation to the principles of causality and sufficient reason, *Leibniz* found it necessary to introduce the principle of the labyrinth. In summary, *Leibniz* has generally been recognized as a profound and versatile student of scientific and philosophical problems in the broadest sense, but many of his ideas seem hopelessly outdated in the 20th century. This is because some of his metaphysical presuppositions are no longer credible. They fail to satisfy many of the criteria later established by *Kant* in the *Critique of Pure Reason* and in the *Critique of Practical Reason.* In our own time, both *Leibniz* and *Kant* seem to be rather deficient in their understanding of essentially anthropological and anthropocentric origins of human beliefs in such questions as teleology, the basis of morality, religion, and ethics.

It should be pointed out that the science of anthropology was not recognized as a genuine scientific discipline until about 1840. It did not begin to develop until the time of *Darwin* and *Huxley,* and to attain maturity until fairly late in the 20th century. At the present time, our thoughts concerning causality must recognize the basis or origins in anthropocentric behavior rather than in metaphysical or critical principles, as understood by *Leibniz* or by *Kant.* These anthropological principles have been grasped more quickly in the English tradition of empiricism than in continental metaphysics of any school or period.

Human Activities of Leibniz

In order better to understand the relevance of *Leibniz* to the philosophy and scientific thought of later times, it is necessary to consider various aspects of his versatile views. According to *Voltaire:* 'In intellectual achievements he was perhaps the most erudite man in Europe: a historian unwearying in documentary research and a profound jurisconsult, illuminating by philosophy alone the study of law, to the practice of which he was apparently a total stranger; a metaphysician so accomplished that he could dispute with the great Newton the invention of the infinitesimal calculus and leave their rivalries a long time doubtful' (*Carr*, 1960).

Leibniz is remembered today as a philosopher, but to understand his relation to *Descartes, Locke, Kant,* and *Newton,* it is necessary to consider some of these other aspects of his life. The turbulent political and religious events of the 17th and 18th centuries coincided with *Leibniz'* career for he was the consultant and adviser of princes as well as the practicing diplomatist. The period witnessed the brilliant reign of Louis XIV, the revolution of 1688 in England, with the rise of the House of Hanover, and the growth of Protestant strength in Holland and elsewhere. It also witnessed the enforced presence of *Locke* in Paris for political reasons.

In this period of *Leibniz'* life about 1690, an important event in European intellectual history occurred — the publication of *Bayle*'s *Dictionary.* This thinker had led a rather erratic religious life, his views oscillating for many years between Catholic and Protestant principles. At the period in question, *Bayle* had arrived at an un-Christian position, accepting the Manichean doctrine of the existence of cosmic evil. According to his metaphysical principle of cosmic optimism, *Leibniz* felt compelled to support his own teleological position. He died in 1744 at the age of 70, but published his religious and metaphysical views in 1711. This was in the form of an extended treatise, *Theodicée,* published in reply to the challenge of *Bayle*'s doctrines.

However, at the beginning of the 18th century, metaphysical doctrines of this kind were practically obsolete. Nevertheless, teleological views continue to survive in many branches of the biomedical sciences, which continue to manifest signs of vitalism (*Joseph,* 1973). Metaphysics of the *Leibniz* type finally were challenged by *Kant,* and failed ultimately to survive his critical philosophy.

Regarding the survival value of Leibnizian and Kantian views in the 20th century, it is possible to cite the authority of so eminent a scientist as *Einstein* (*Born-Einstein,* 1971). In a letter written to *Max Born* dated September 15, 1950, *Einstein* wrote ... 'I see from the last paragraph of your letter that you, too, take the quantum theoretical description as incomplete (referring to the ensemble). But you are after all convinced that no (complete) laws exist for a complete description, according to the positivistic maxim *(esse est percipii).* Well, this is a programmatic attitude, not knowledge. This is where our attitudes really differ. For the time being, I am alone in my views as *Leibniz* was with respect to the absolute space of *Newton*'s theory.'

In his commentary on this passage, *Born* wrote: 'This is probably the clearest presentation of *Einstein*'s philosophy of reality ... an exact description of the state of a physical system presupposes that one can make statements of infinite precision about it.'

To *Born* this seems absurd. However, in our time, no one can doubt that *Leibniz* must have been skeptical toward the Newtonian (and Cartesian) ideas as to the reality of absolute space and time. Both must have regarded *motion, process,* or *event* as the ultimate realities. Thus, the conception of *Einstein* and of *Leibniz* have definitely prevailed in the 20th century (*Whitehead,* 1925, 1929).

In relation to the views of *Kant* regarding causality, *Einstein* at one point compared them with those of the English empiricists, as represented by *Hume.* In an undated letter to *Born, Einstein* wrote as follows: 'I am reading *Kant*'s *Prologomena* here among other things, and am beginning to comprehend the enormous suggestive power that emanated from the fellow, and still does. Once you concede to him merely the existence of synthetic *a priori* judgements, you are trapped. I have to water down the *a priori* to 'conventional', so as not to have to contradict him, but even then, the details do not fit. Anyway, it is very nice to read, even if it is not as good as his predecessor *Hume*'s work. *Hume* also had a far sounder instinct.'

It seems clear from this brief passage that *Einstein* must have shared the skepticism that both *Locke* and *Hume* felt toward synthetic *a priori* judgements concerning causality. This skepticism would also be consonant with *Leibniz*' views as to the nature of the 'labyrinth'.

Principle of Sufficient Reason

In the year 1813, almost exactly a century after the death of *Leibniz,* the philosopher *Schopenhauer* published his essay *The Fourfold Root of the Principle of Sufficient Reason.* By this principle, he meant the truism that there is a reason, or cause for any given fact or existent entity. 'Nothing is without a reason for its being.' Thus, everything in nature is in relation to something else. This has usually been regarded by philosophers and scientists to be self-evident and to require no proof. *Schopenhauer* recognized not one but *four* such principles: physical, logical, mathematical and moral.

If each given thing, or object, in a given physical or biological system is related or explicable in connection to some other existent, then there must be an elaborate chain of causality that connects all the parts of such a system. In modern science, such systems are usually treated by statistical methods. In physics and chemistry, the science of statistical mechanics is applied. In human and animal biology, the related sciences may be those of 'vital statistics' or of 'mathematical biology'. Here the tendency is not to regard any given vital phenomenon as dependent on the simple location of each material particle in a given macroscopic assembly, but to treat the whole system as a unified entity. One such abstract theoretical method is that of thermodynamics, based on *Carnot*'s principle and on *Gibbs' Equilibrium of Heterogeneous Substances,* or the phase rule (*Joseph,* 1971a, b; 1973).

When the biological system or an ecological system is *open and restricted,* it is possible to treat it by the methods of physical biology, as based on physical laws in each of an infinite number of steps.

In the previously mentioned *Born-Einstein Letters* (1950), *Born* comments in relation to *Einstein*'s views: '... an exact description of the state of a physical system presupposes that one can make statements of infinite precision about it.' In modern physics, such attempts are rarely made. In other words, the principle of sufficient reason gives way to one of statistical law, or to a law of probability. What is true of the physical sciences holds also for biological sciences. Thus, in a complex human society of millions of individuals, human behavior is not generally referred to this or that individual man, woman or child, but is referred to norms for the population as a whole, or for given sections of it. Thus, the whole science of demography, for example, is treated on the basis of statistical probability rather than by any principle of sufficient reason, as applied to each given unit of the population. In this way, one avoids a labyrinth, previously described by *Leibniz* (1765).

One of the labyrinths treated by *Leibniz* in the *Theodicée:* 'consists in the discussion *of continuity and of the indivisibles* which appear to be the elements of it into which the consideration of *infinity* must enter'. This labyrinth does not trouble or embarass those who apply only reasoning based on the principles of *Clausius-Carnot, Gibbs,* or *Claude Bernard,* which is free of the fallacies of the labyrinth: causal connections need not be referred to the principle of sufficient reason.

On the other hand, biological systems studied by Cartesian or Newtonian notions of reality have often been based on the actual positions of infinite assemblies of particles in space and time, and require explanations based on an infinity of cause-effect relations between individual and indivisible units or elements which enter into a continuum. Thus, mechanistic explanations in the biological sciences, including physiology, involve a labyrinth of causal steps. One emerges from the labyrinth only by the methods of *Carnot, Gibbs,* and *Claude Bernard (Joseph,* 1973).

Law and Causality in Biology

To the groups of English skeptical empiricists who were primarily interested in human nature must be added the 19th and 20th century followers of *Carnot, Helmholtz, Joule,* and *Mayer* in the physical sciences. Thus, 'the principle of causality is nothing else but the supposition that all the phenomena of nature are subject to law' *(von Helmholtz). Joule* (1847) regarded living force, *vis viva,* as a property natural to all bodies ... 'as such, it would be absurd to suppose that it can be destroyed'. Thus, according to the first law of thermodynamics, the principle of causality is fully replaced by that of a law of conservation. That this is applicable to living animals, including man, was fully understood in the 19th and 20th centuries *(Benedict and Cathcart,* 1913; *Catchpole and Joseph,* 1974).

It is clear that *Claude Bernard* clearly understood the principles of law and causality in comparative biology and physiology. Thus, in 1856 he wrote: 'We seek the laws of phenomena, that is to say, whatever is stable, invariable, permanent, and eternal in these phenomena ... In the immense variety of objects that surround us we thus look for what is invariable: the law.' In any science, the principle of law expresses itself through the regular recurrence of invariant objects associated with invariant phenomena. Thus, the concept of cause and effect is no longer required and can be replaced by a law of nature. Hence, according to *Whitehead* (1925), 'It is unnecessary to labor the point, that in broad outline certain general states of nature recur, and that our very natures have adapted themselves to such repetitions. But there is a complementary fact which is equally true and equally obvious — nothing really recurs in exact detail. No two days are identical, no two winters. The details emanate 'from the inscrutable womb of things beyond the ken of rationality. Men expected the sun to arise, but the wind bloweth where it listeth'.

Accordingly, astronomy and other branches of cosmology are exact Newtonian or Einsteinian sciences, but the phenomena of meteorology (the science of weather) are subject to rather unpredictable vagaries. The data of meteorology cannot be expressed by exact scientific law. Thus, the forces and causes (wind, barometric pressures, temperatures, and rainfall) may be expressed only by average values, with rather considerable statistical deviations. Human and animal behavior, insofar as they depend on meteorology and climatology, cannot be exactly predictable. Thus, all the behavioral sciences must be regarded as conforming to principles of immediate causality governed by statistical interrelations among many complex variable forces. In these fields, generalizations are entirely inductive and subject, in great measure to skepticism of the Humean kind (chapter 5).

Anthropological and Ethological Behavior

The principle of sufficient reason was perhaps best understood during the period from *Leibniz* to *Schopenhauer*, because, as explained in the foregoing, it was approached from the point of view of anthropological and anthropocentric phenomenology and behavior, although these terms were not used at the time. In the physical sciences, the principle was replaced by the followers of *Newton* and by those of *Carnot, von Helmholtz, Joule,* and *Mayer.* As we have seen in the preceding pages, the concept of law, as developed by *Claude Bernard* in the science of general physiology, was related to a principle of invariance or homeostasis. Invariance can be easily understood in relation to *Carnot*'s principle when expressed as the concept of *Conservation of Reversibility* (*Joseph,* 1973).

From the point of view of the principle of *Carnot-Clausius,* it is convenient to classify any biological process as either reversible or irreversible. Invariant conditions within the organism, such as the maintenance of constant electrolyte composition, constant water balance, constant freezing point, and acid-base balance in all phases of the heterogeneous system, are explained by *Gibbs*' phase rule as an aspect of the 'equilibrium of heterogeneous substances' (*Gibbs,* 1875, 1928). Irreversible processes such as growth, development and aging of various cells and tissues are then classed along with respiratory metabolism as *irreversible* processes. These distinctions apply to the resting or standard state of any type of cell or tissue during periods of phylogenetic and ontogenetic development. The most constant properties are the chemical potentials of water and electrolytes in the fluid phases of the *milieu interieur* (*Joseph,* 1971a, b, 1973). The electrolyte composition of these phases also tend to remain constant, implying invariant standard conditions (*Macallum,* 1910, 1926). However, at *constant chemical potentials* of water and *inorganic electrolytes* in the solid or semi-solid phases of many cells and tissues, the ionic concentrations depend on the *standard chemical potentials* of the several ions (Na, K, Ca, Mg, Cl). These are dielectric properties that depend on the state of aggregation of each phase (*Joseph,* 1971a, b, 1973). These properties can be observed or calculated by various methods, and have been shown to be related to the mean ionic radii (*Born,* 1920; *Laidler and Pegis,* 1957).

Behavioral processes, involving changes in configurational entropy and free energy of irritable or contractile properties of neuromuscular tissues and of the various sensory organs, are therefore related to the dielectric properties of water in various labile states of aggregation (*Joseph,* 1971a, b, 1973; *Catchpole and Joseph,* 1974). Accordingly, behavior and chemical morphology both depend on labile states of aggregation (*Joseph,* 1971a, b, 1973). Hence human or animal behavior (ethology) may be classed under the subject of chemical morphology, and its changes of state, as described by water-electrolyte composition, chemical and electrical potentials.

Physical or structural anthropology then depends on species, age, and development, as described by the *laws* of phylogeny, ontogeny, and genetics. These are laws which are contingent in relation to time development and the composition of the cosmic environment. They are *necessary* in relation to the genes and chromosomes, which determine speciation.

Behavior then depends on certain fixed conditions in organism and environment (speciation, physical biology, and respiratory metabolism). However, it also depends on various factors related to adaptation or 'fitness'. Thus, the behavior of human beings depends on professional or occupational training (musician, actor, hunter or farmer). This is true also of animal behavior (hunting dogs, police dogs, work dogs, and so forth). The behavior of men and animals thus follows principles of law (morphology and species), as well as principles of sufficient reason (ethics, morals, specific duties). These depend on anthropological or ethological factors in human or animal behavior. Physical, structural and chemical anthropology would, on the contrary, depend entirely on species. Then, as explained by *Locke,* behavior is *a postiori,* and determined by processes of empirical education or training. Contrary to Lamarckian views, it is not *innate* or *congenital.* Thus, the theories of *Darwin* and *Huxley* are consonant with the views of modern biologists, who reject the principles of Lamarckism, as opposed to Mendelian biology.

Ethological behavior is, of course, greatly conditioned by geophysical, geochemical, and meteorological conditions. The hours of sunrise and sunset determine recurrent geophysical conditions of illumination and temperature, which must certainly be imposed on the 'instincts' and behavior of all mammals, including man. Thus, all species adopt more or less regular habits of feeding and hours of arising and retiring. These regular meteorological features are recurrent and subject to the whims of nature, which may be quite inseparable. At various times and places of human history, these inseparable forces may be very mysterious. This gives rise to fear, anxiety, and mystery, to superstition and irrational behavior in savage and other untutored human societies. Conceptions of scientific law may be absent in primitive societies.

Chapter 7

Voluntarism

The principles of scientific knowledge depend on the acquisition of empirical sense-data, on the formulation of the principles of causality and law, and on the rational study of human nature as the basis of constitutional law and moral behavior (chapters 4 and 5). These principles of human understanding were among the great motives of the 18th century enlightenment in Europe. By the time of *Kant*, the philosophy of the English empiricists, *Locke* and *Hume*, had definitely established sensation, perception, and understanding as the basis of enlightened human behavior, not only in science, but also in the philosophy of government, law, and human affairs. Especially in England and France, this was the period in which is found the transition from the medieval world of feudalism and scholasticism to the world of modern science and philosophy.

In science, the period witnessed the transition from Newtonian mechanics and the Cartesian method to the generalized principles of energy and entropy, as expressed by *Sadi Carnot* in thermodynamics. The corresponding development in philosophy was that of metaphysics as understood by *Leibniz* to the later period of *Kant*'s critical philosophy. At that time, the question of the relation of necessary to contingent laws was scrutinized. The principles of induction were critically studied, and the basis of certainty in science was sought in a universal order of nature. This was based on Newtonian physics and a generalized kind of mathematics. The equations of mathematical physics became highly abstract; the results became independent of the nature of any particular entity or class of entities. Thus, the generalized equations of physics applied equally well to mechanics, optics, acoustics, and finally to electricity and magnetism.

In the development of science from *Newton* to *Kant*, there was no place for voluntarism. This is an anthropomorphic conception, and the main object of physical science was to conceive of a physical universe of eternal objects in which man was pictured as an impartial observer. Nature was thought to be governed by permanent laws that remain independent of the nature of any given entity or set of entities. The order of nature, so conceived, also remains indifferent to human desires, feelings, and emotions. In the limit, the ideal of physical law became completely abstract, mathematical, and independent of all anthropocentric values. Thus, by its nature, physics was compelled to exclude any element of voluntarism or of human will.

The English empiricists, *Locke* and *Hume*, however, had taught that all human understanding was based on ideas that enter consciousness through the sense organs. This conception of science implied that all human ideas were to that extant *a postiori* and dependent on the nature of the thought process. Thought is communicated by speech and language. These begin in the neuromuscular system, and are developed by processes of human history and social life. Our belief in an order of nature thus depends on the validity of the principles of induction *(Hume)* and on anthropocentric interpretations of law and causality. Thus, the issues raised by *Leibniz* and *Kant* seem ultimately to have been resolved in favor of the English empiricists (*Born-Einstein Letters*, 1971).

These views are involved in the general philosophical questions of voluntarism. The questions came to the foreground in German philosophy of the 19th century, particularly as expressed by *Schopenhauer* (1788–1860) and *Nietzsche* (1844–1900).

Will and Idea

The philosophy of *Schopenhauer* acknowledges his indebtedness not only to *Plato* and *Aristotle* among the ancients, but also to *Leibniz* and *Kant* among his more immediate predecessors. His most important early work was *The Fourfold Root of the Principle of Sufficient Reason* (1813). This was followed by *The World as Will and Idea* (1818), with second and third editions following in 1844 and 1860, respectively. The third edition, completed at the age of 72, shows the fecundity of *Schopenhauer*'s conception of *will*, which is applied to all aspects of human reason, including aesthetics, morality, and ethics. The concept was also applied to all forms of life, which necessarily manifest *will*, as well as perception, knowledge and ideas.

Schopenhauer regards some forms of reason as necessary and *a priori*. In this, he agrees with *Plato* and *Kant*. Thus, the principle of *causality* and that of *sufficient reason* are regarded as self-evident and transcendent rather than empirical. Following *Plato*, he regarded the existent objective world to enter human consciousness in two different forms: homogeneous classes of universals, and second, as specific, distinct identifiable particular entities. Science, according to *Schopenhauer*, required classification of all its data, originating in the phenomenological external world into these two classes: the general and the specific. The principles of biology, for example, are then transcendental and *a priori*. This is required by the principle of sufficient reason, which requires that every object of our sense perceptions must have a *cause* (chapter 6).

It was also recognized by *Schopenhauer* that the objectivization of the *Will* in the animal or human organism required *self-presentation* and self-exhibition in the 'real corporeal world'. In higher organisms, this depends on the organization of the brain and central nervous system. The necessary condition for this is the existence of the body as an anatomical and morphological entity. This is an *existence;* any attributes of the body, including *will,* is an *essence.* Philosophers have always divided themselves into two main groups: (1) existentialists or phenomenologists, and (2) transcendalists, subjective idealists, or those who emphasize *essence.* The first group can be exemplified by *Aristotle* and all the predecessors of empirical science. In the second group are to be found *Plato, Pythagoras,* and the ancient Hebrew prophets.

Although *Schopenhauer* believed that animal will and behavior required the animal body and brain, he was fully aware that these essences were permanent and fundamental. He quotes experiments by *Spallanzani* and by *Voltaire,* showing that invertebrates recover their normal perceptions and behavior after removal or excision of various parts of the body. Regeneration of animal or human cells and tissues after injury or surgery are phenomena that are so familiar that they require no detailed discussion. After such serious operations as removal of vital organs, such as a lung or a kidney, most human beings undergo no permanent or irreversible changes in the *will. Schopenhauer* related this to the *will to live* or the *will to believe.* This essence can be related to *Kant*'s 'thing in itself' rather than to the perception or description of the world of external objects (the *idea*). Evidently, we may believe that this human *essence* is the most enduring and permanent quality of any living being in either the world of human beings or in that of any biological species. It can never be completely separated from material existence, which in biology presupposes living protoplasm. This in turn depends on the invariance of the structure of the genes and chromosomes (*Schrodinger,* 1944; *Joseph,* 1973). There is an element of chance in the time required for the various kinds of structural changes that can occur in the macromolecular structure of a gene. The time required for a given kind of mutation increases exponentially with the excitation energy required to activate the mutation. Thus:

$$t = \text{constant} \times \exp \frac{W}{kT},$$

where W is the 'activation energy', k is the *Boltzmann* constant, and T is the absolute temperature. Stability is measured by t, the 'expectation period' of a given mutation. Some typical values of t and W are as follows:

Expectation time, t	W, eV	Type of radiation
0.1 sec	0.9	infrared
16 months	1.5	visible
30,000 years	11.8	visible
1 million years	13.2	X-rays
100 million years	20.0	hard X-rays

Many biological species have existed in geological time for periods of more than 100 million years. These include certain arthropods, brachiopods, and crustaceans. Such species would be able to resist the effects of very powerful ionizing radiations, such as hard X-rays and gamma rays.

Expressing this property of long survival, it could be said that such very stable species are characterized by the power of their 'will to live'. This power also applies to the essence of any such species, which retains its permanence with respect to perceptions, 'irritability', responses to stimuli, and ecological behavior.

All protoplasm manifests specific properties of 'irritability', or the ability to respond to stimuli (*Glisson*, 1650; *von Haller*, 1753; *Peirce*, 1892; *Joseph*, 1973; *Catchpole and Joseph*, 1974). This property may be considered to depend on the existence of protoplasmic water in two or more labile states of aggregation (*Stensen*, 1664; *Peirce*, 1892; *Joseph*, 1973; *Catchpole and Joseph*, 1974). Thus, *Schopenhauer*'s concept of *'Will'* or *Kant*'s concept of 'thing in itself' may be ultimately related to changes of state of water in given kinds of sensory or motor nerves.

Irritability of Protoplasm

To approach the problem of the existence and essence of any given type of protoplasm, it is necessary to consider the historical point of view. A brief historical outline from the point of view of the cell theory is available (*Joseph*, 1973).

The cell theory of *Schleiden and Schwann* (*Schleiden*, 1842; *Schwann*, 1839) was to a large extent the culmination of the earlier microscopic observations of protoplasm dating from the studies of *von Rosenhof* (1753) on the ameba. Other kinds of protoplasmic movement in plant cells were observed and described by *Brown* (1825). The sensitivity and delicacy of these movements are indicated by the discovery of the microscopic 'Brownian movement'. The physical basis of these observations was not well understood until the 20th century, when it was finally explained by *Einstein*'s theory of the kinetic energy and motion of colloidal particles (1905–1908).

The theory of Schleiden and Schwann appeared at about the same time as the concept of 'protoplasm'. This term seems to have been used for the first time by *Purkinje* (1825) to denote the substance that is first formed by the cell. It is derived from two Greek words ('protos' = first) and ('plasma' = formed substance). The term was widely used with various connotations by numerous biologists and histologists (*von Rosenhof*, 1753; *von Mohl*, 1871; *Schultze*, 1863; *Minchin*, 1912).

In 1868, *Thomas Huxley* expressed the following opinion '... that the dull vital actions of a fungus or a foraminifer are the properties of their protoplasm, and are the direct results of the matter of which they are composed ... (and) it must be said to be the result of the molecular forces of the protoplasm which displays it'. It would follow from *Huxley*'s opinion that 'will and idea' are inherent in the structure and behavior of protoplasm.

Writing nearly a century later, *Frey-Wyssling* (1953) expressed his opinion that: 'It is therefore out of the question that any living constituent of protoplasm could consist of structureless, fluid, independently displaceable particles.' From the biological point of view, will, purpose, ideas and perceptions depend on the chemical morphology of protoplasm and the 'life slimes' in the neuromuscular system, the brain, the sense organs, and in the *milieu intérieur*. The 'will to live' and the 'will to believe' are, from this point of view, enduring properties that depend on the genetic stability of each kind of species.

The Primitive Nervous System

From what has been said, it would not have been possible to develop the study of the nervous system from the point of view of chemical morphology, histology, or histochemistry, independently of the subject of cytology at microscopic and submicroscopic levels (*Joseph,* 1973). Thus, the phenomenology of behavior depends on the results of physical and structural anthropology in the broadest sense. This opinion seems to be shared by *Frey-Wyssling* (1953), who concludes his book *Submicroscopic Morphology of Protoplasm* with the motto *Structura omnis e Structura.*

Classification of any anatomical structure or unit with reference to the subsets of structures at cellular levels is necessary in the determination of its behavior. This always requires an understanding of its nature as a purposeful, well-ordered and heterogeneous physicochemical system. A theory of the physicochemical behavior of intracellular phases of protoplasm (nucleus and cytoplasm) first of all requires the development of appropriate techniques of histology and histochemistry at microscopic and submicroscopic levels. At the present time, many such methods have been developed in the fields of visible, ultraviolet and infrared microscopy, the use of polarized light, and in studies of X-ray diffraction and electron microscopy. Optical techniques of many kinds are now available; these can be applied to a great variety of problems.

As has been pointed out, the cell theory was initiated about 1840. The development of exact histological and cytochemical methods was essential to the application of the theory to all problems relating to the morphology and behavior of any part of the central or autonomic systems. An understanding of morphology was therefore requisite to the comprehension of neuromuscular irritability and responsiveness, as well as of their relations to sense perception, knowledge, and will. To a large extent, these functions are dependent on phylogenetic development; they are well-developed in the higher vertebrates (mammals and birds), but remain poorly developed in cold blooded vertebrates and invertebrates. Thus, *Schopenhauer*'s 'will and idea' require the coordination of all parts of a highly evolved, well-ordered and purposeful neuromuscular system. In primitive organisms, the concept of voluntarism tends to vanish. Survival then depends only to a slight extent on any discernable 'will to live', 'will to power', or 'survival of the fittest'. It depends only on the stability of the genes, resulting from their high activation energies with respect to the formation of mutant isomers. Activation energies and the expectation times of isomer formation may be especially high in such invertebrates as arthropods, crustaceans, and molluscs. The tempo and mode of evolution are thus to a great extent biological indications of a 'will to live'. This is a primary property of existence, which implies the nature of all secondary properties related to 'essence': behavior, ideas, and voluntarism.

In the more primitive invertebrates, contractility and irritability of myofibrils and other contractile elements are stimulated directly by environmental changes, and require no innervation by any other kind of conducting fibers (*Parker*, 1918). This generalization applies to organisms such as sponges, which are at a lower phylogenetic level than that of the coelenterates (jelly fish and sea anemones, for example).

In response to changes of salinity or other conditions of the environmental sea water, sponges are able to produce flow of liquid through surface pores by way of a system of internal canals that lead to a circular *osculum*. by alternate contractions and extensions, this muscular tissue is able to control the passage of liquid from the interior canals to the environmental sea water, thus regulating the volume and hydrostatic pressure within the organism. At this level of invertebrate evolution, nervous control of muscular irritability is neither required nor observed.

Various kinds of muscular contraction in higher vertebrates such as mammals likewise require no nervous stimulation. This is true, for example, of the optical iris, in which contraction can be induced by intense visible light impinging on the eye. Thus, certain types of muscle can contract in response to direct stimulation by light (*Parker*, 1918), whereas others respond directly to changes of environmental salinity, chemical composition, hydrostatic pressure, electrical currents, or to a gravitational field. These responses are usually called 'tropisms'. They are classified according to the nature of the stimulus: phototropism, galvanotropism, geotropisms, or chemotropisms. Familiar examples of phototropism are the responses of moths or other insects to visible light or the attraction of the sunflower toward solar illumination. Thus, plants as well as animals exhibit many examples of various tropisms. Although subject to certain doubts at the time, the contractility of the denervated iris in response to light observed in the eye of such vertebrates as frogs and eels in the early years of the 20th century seems to have been confirmed under various experimental conditions (*Parker,* 1918). Muscular irritability and contractility in such cases would seem to imply related changes in the state of intrafibrillar water (*Joseph,* 1973).

In direct responses of tissues to external stimuli, the organism exhibits little or no evidence of any *will* or *idea.* The tissue response or tropism has generally been regarded as a 'forced movement beyond the will, control or volition of the animal or plant'. It would be safe to suppose that *'will* and *idea or representation'* imply the reception of external stimuli by sensory nerve endings and the transmission of afferent nerve impulses through a ganglion or 'center' to nerve endings in an effector organ (muscle fiber, secretory gland, or other type of *effector*). Thus, the most primitive type of reflex arc would be typified by the scheme:

$$\text{Stimulus} \xrightarrow{\dfrac{\text{afferent fiber}}{\text{receptor}}} \text{center} \xrightarrow{\dfrac{\text{efferent fiber}}{\text{motor neurone}}} \text{Effector.}$$

According to *Schopenhauer* and his metaphysical predecessors of the 18th and 19th centuries, ideas and understanding are related to sensation and perception in the following way. The process of perception requires not only the reception of a given type of sensation (visible, auditory, or tactile), but also the understanding of the *nature* of the object. This is an *idea* present in the mind through previous *a postiori* empirical experience. Thus, a child obtains a visual impression of an object such as a chair or a table; *perception* of the object is an act of *understanding* at which he arrives only through experience. He can then place the chair at its proper place in order to consume his lunch. This is an act of *will.* Thus, corresponding to the diagram of the primitive reflex arc, the following scheme can be shown:

(1)	(2)	(3)	(4)	(5)
Visual stimulus	→ Sensation	→ Perception of idea	→ Act of will	→ Consumption of food

This illustrates a fundamental fact of general physiology: sensation, perception, and volition are coordinated and integrated in ganglionic centers in the cerebral cortex. This coordination occurs in steps 2, 3, and 4 of the above scheme. Stimulation occurs in nerve endings of the receptor (eye, ear, skin). Sensation occurs in the cortical center, where it is coordinated with will and idea by an integrative process.

Ideas are related to previously existing empirical knowledge according to the principles of *knowledge* and *language,* as enunciated by *Locke* (chapter 4). *Will* or *volition* is a result of a purposeful decision formulated by the entire brain, acting as a unit. This decision is executed by efferent (motor) nerves that activate the requisite sets of skeletal muscles, and integrated with coordinated nerves of the autonomic system. Thus, many kinds and sets of afferent and efferent nerves are required to activate or inhibit many different kinds and sets of skeletal and smooth muscle. The investigation of the microscopic and sub-microscopic structures includes the study of neuroplasm and of cytoplasm in general, and has continued for considerably more than a century.

Neuroplasm

No systematic investigation of the histology, histochemistry, or chemical morphology of the central nervous system of the higher vertebrates, including man, would have been possible in the early years of the 19th century. Such studies necessarily would have required the general principles of cytology, as it depends on the cell theory of *Schleiden and Schwann* and on the concomitant investigations of protoplasm, as defined by *Purkinje* (1825), *von Mohl* (1871) and subsequent investigators.

As early as 1842, *von Helmholtz* showed the presence in invertebrates of fibrous elements in the nervous system, and also demonstrated their relationship to structures later known as ganglion cells. *Kolliker* (1885) showed a similar relationship between myelinated fibers and ganglia. It is interesting that these early observations of fibers and ganglia were published simultaneously with the second edition of *Schopenhauer*'s *The World as Will and Representation.* A relationship between these purely philosophical reflections and the scientific study of the vertebrate brain and nervous system has been established in the preceding section of this chapter (Primitive Innervation).

After these early studies, it was necessary to establish the morphological relationships between fibrous elements and the corpuscular ganglia in all parts of the nervous system. To these two constituents of the central nervous system of vertebrates, it was later necessary to add a third — the gray matter. On microscopic examination, the gray matter was shown to have the appearance of very fine points rather than that of a continuum. After about 1850, it was therefore designated as 'punctate substance'. After the introduction of the Golgi method of staining by means of silver impregnation, more precise histochemical studies became possible. Finally, in 1891, it was shown by *Kolliker* that at some point every nerve fiber is connected with a ganglion cell. It should be noted that this observation can be dated about 50 years subsequent to the observations of *von Helmholtz* in 1842 and the cell theory of *Schleiden and Schwann* in 1839/1842.

Late in the 19th century, it was finally recognized that what was first termed the ganglion cell was in fact the nucleated body of the neurone, which is the true nerve cell.

From the nucleated body, two types of processes emanate: (1) fine protoplasmic processes, and (2) gray matter, or punctate substance. Neighboring neurones may possibly be connected by gray matter.

Embryological studies have shown that in the earliest stages of development, the *neuroplasts* were rather widely separated. The fully developed neurone could be observed at a later stage of embryonic development to approach neighboring neurones in the same state. This process was necessary to permit the transmission of nerve impulses from the ganglion cell to the branched nerve endings. Thus, integrated organization of a completed reflex arc depends on processes of growth and development. Development of 'will and idea', or of perception, understanding and volition is, as we would expect, a function of age and development of the central nervous system. Behavior (or *will*) can never be completely separated from morphological development during the growth period of mammals, although in later life they may tend to become independent. This would tend to support *Locke*'s arguments against the existence of innate ideas, rather than *Kant*'s belief in the possibility of certain kinds of synthetic *a priori* judgements (chapters 4 and 6).

Spinal Reflexes

Bodily reactions in general are governed by motor fibers in the central nervous system which terminate in peripheral motor nerves and *synapses* in all parts of the nervous systems; connections between different nerve fibers, or between nerve and muscle require the presence of intervening structures known as 'synapses'. Thus, for the body as a whole, two main types of controls may be distinguished: (1) voluntary controls coordinated by motor fibers in the cerebral cortex, as they are influenced by sensory fibers originating in various peripheral regions of the body, and (2) the unit motor and sensory fibers in the spinal cord in the simple reflex. This is the basis of neuromuscular stimulation and contraction, flexion, extension and tension. The sensory and motor fibers in any given unit are coordinated to provide integrated and purposeful behavior in many reflex arcs in the peripheral neuromuscular system of any given mammalian species.

In the 'spinal dog', for example, various simple reflex arcs have been identified as unit processes. These include the 'reflexor reflex' and the 'scratch reflex', each of which has been studied in great detail by *Sherrington* (1920). Comparable reflexes in man are the 'knee jerk' and the 'flexor' reflexes. Normally, these responses of protoplasm to voluntary controls occur in both sets of neuromuscular and sensory fibers.

Dielectric Properties of Nerve

The following properties of intermuscular or of nervous protoplasm are related to the dielectric constant, D'': the standard chemical potential of each kind of inorganic physiological ion, the action potential, E_a, the resting potential, E, the dielectric energy, $c_{Na}'' \Delta\mu_{Na}°$, and (for skeletal muscle), the maximal work and isometric tension. The following relations, among others, have been developed (*Joseph*, 1971a, b; 1973; chapter 3 of the preceding treatment):

$$\Delta\mu_{Na}° = \frac{164}{b_{Na}} \left(\frac{1}{D''} - \frac{1}{80} \right)$$

(change of standard chemical potential of Na ion),

$E_a = 43.4 \ \Delta\mu_{Na}°$
(action potential in mV; $\Delta\mu_{Na}°$ in kcal),

Maximal work = $c_{Na}'' \ \Delta\mu_{Na}°$
(maximal work is equal to the dielectric energy measured in calories or joules).

Tension = $8.6 \ c_{Na}'' \ \Delta\mu_{Na}°$

Thus, from measurements of the action potential, it is possible to obtain values of $\Delta\mu_{Na}°$ and D''. The value of b_{Na}, the corrected ionic radius is taken as 1.25 Å units.

The values of the above parameters can also be calculated from the intracellular and extracellular electrolyte concentrations (*Joseph*, 1973). The method is applicable to neuroplasm as well as the myoplasm. The following values have been calculated for the following kinds of nerve tissue, using values of E_a given by *Hodgkin* (1951):

Tissue	E_a, mV	$\Delta\mu_{Na}°$, kcal	Dielectric constant D''
Loligo axon	90[1]	2.08	35
Loligo axon	88[1]	2.03	35
Loligo axon	104[1]	2.39	32
Sepia axon	120[1]	2.74	30
Sepia axon	124[1]	2.85	29
Frog neurone	116	2.70	30

[1] Squid.

Thus, the values of D'' for neuroplasm range from 29 to 35 for the squid axon, corresponding to values of from 2.03 to 2.85 kcal for the change of standard chemical potential of sodium. Values of 2.70–2.80 kcal and values of

D'' of about 30 are characteristic of mammalian and frog skeletal muscle as well as of frog nerve. Thus, muscle and nerve preparations of various kinds may show similar values of D'' and $\Delta\mu_{Na}^{\circ}$, indicating rather similar states of aggregation and free energies of hydration, in structures that differ greatly with respect to function. In every case, stimulation results in production of the action potential, E_a, corresponding to a change of state of the protoplasm from D'' to a value in the neighborhood of 80, as for pure water. The value of the free energy of hydration of the sodium ion in pure water or in the stimulated myofibril is about 164 kcal/mole of sodium. In the unstimulated or resting state of the myofibril, the value is about 161.2 kcal/mole. The difference (164−161.2), or 2.8 kcal, is the difference of free energy of hydration between the extracellular and intracellular phases, or between the stimulated and resting states. The conversion factor between kcal and millivolts is 43.4 mV/kcal. Thus, a value of 2.80 kcal for $\Delta\mu_{Na}^{\circ}$ corresponds to a calculated action potential of about 122 mV. When the free energy of sodium in pure water is assumed to be 164 kcal, as referred to a state of vacuum, in which the dielectric constant is 1.0, then the resting intrafibrillar state implies a hydration energy of 161.2 kcal. This accounts for the property of intracellular water to have a relatively low concentration of sodium − the transfer of the ion to a medium of low dielectric constant increases the free energy of hydration by 2.8 kcal/mole, corresponding to an action potential of about 120 mV. Thus the source of energy for muscular contraction or for the conduction of nervous impulses resides in the relatively high hydration energy of the structured intracellular water, as referred to the stimulated state.

Comparable values of $\Delta\mu_{Na}^{\circ}$, D'' and dielectric energy for human whole brain have been estimated from analytical data (*Widdowson and Dickerson, 1964*):

	$\Delta\mu_{Na}^{\circ}$, kcal	$c_{Na}''\,\Delta\mu_{Na}^{\circ}$, cal/kg water	D''
Whole brain	0.70	50.05	58
White matter	0.51	49.60	61
Gray matter	0.56	51.30	59

The values of D'' for brain are about 60; this agrees with earlier results for various mammals (*Joseph*, 1971a, b; 1973). The change of standard chemical potential of sodium is small (0.51−0.70 kcal), and the dielectric energy is about 50 cal/kg water. Since the adult human brain contains about 1 kg water, the dielectric energy of whole brain is about 50 cal, distributed among about 10 billion neurones. Thus, each neurone contains on the average about 10^{-7} g of water, with a dielectric energy content of 5×10^{-9} cal.

In a man of 70 kg weight, the brain weighs about 1.3 kg, as compared with about 30 kg for the total weight of skeletal muscle. Therefore, the following comparison can be made:

	Total weight, kg	Weight of water, kg	Total dielectric energy, cal
Whole brain	1.3	1.0	50
Skeletal muscle	30.1	22.5	1,800

Thus, in a total of 1,850 cal of dielectric energy distributed between brain and skeletal muscle, the proportion in muscle to brain is approximately 36 to 1. This is explained by the fact that the external work of the body is produced by voluntary skeletal muscle; the internal work, dielectric energy and hydration energy of brain, motor nerves, and sense organs are relatively small. The energy transmitted by sensory nerves to the cortical sensory and motor centers is likewise only a small fraction of the total metabolic energy. Thus, by far the greater fraction of metabolic energy (or dielectric energy) is spent in the skeletal muscles, as compared with the central nervous system. As in any well designed machine, energy is used in effecting external work (or locomotion) rather than in the control system or steering mechanisms. The energy is spent as *will;* the control is operated by ideas and *knowledge.* The human caloric requirements are high in the operations of *physical* work — low in sedentary or mental work.

Chapter 8

Monism and Pluralism

Three conceivable ways of explaining the early forms of Cartesian dualism have been described by *Peirce* in *The Structure of Theories* (1892). These were designated as follows to indicate the types of relation between the physical and psychic laws: (a) *Independence:* a doctrine sometimes called *monism*, but preferably *neutralism*. (b) *Materialism,* in which the physical law is primary, and the psychical law of the body is secondary. (c) *Idealism:* the psychical law is primary, and the physical law of the body is secondary.

The second mode of explication, the materialist, is the only method conceivable, if it is granted that all the operations of the body and mind are governed entirely by physical and chemical mechanisms. An early example of this view would be represented by the views of early Cartesians such as *Joseph La Mettrie,* who is an extreme exponent of the view that the living organism is a *machine.* Although this idea has obtained little support in philosophical circles, it has received tacit support from many physiologists and biochemists, who have supported a *vitalist* position in these sciences, as opposed to the *anti-vitalist* or organicist views of such students of bioenergetics as *von Helmholtz, Joule, Mayer, Claude Bernard, Henderson, Cannon,* and *Sherrington. Peirce* himself regarded *materialism* in biology as 'repugnant'; it would derive *thought* from the properties of matter. Non-living matter he considered to be a degraded form of living substance.

According to *Peirce,* the one tenable solution of the problem must necessarily take the form of *objective idealism,* as opposed to the subjective idealism of Bishop *Berkeley* (chapter 5).

Objective idealism, as opposed to subjectivism, agrees with the type of empiricism supported by *Hume* and by his nominalist predecessor, *William of Occam.* Independence of the psychic law and the physical law (monism or neutralism) are condemned by the principle of *Occam*'s razor: 'entities are not to be multiplied without necessity'.

It might be argued that, of all the philosophers from *Descartes* to *Peirce,* the idea of 'objective idealism' is best represented by the 'will and idea' of *Schopenhauer. Idea* represents the psychic aspect of human knowledge. It is *objective* in that it originates in external sense-objects as they enter consciousness by way of the sense organs and sensory nerves. The *psychic* aspect of human consciousness and behavior requires sensation, perception and understanding that depend on the *physical* properties of neuroplasm, chemical morphology, and cytology. Thus, well-ordered human and animal behavior requires a physicochemical coordination between *will and idea,* or between sensation, perception, and volition, as they represent the physical and psychic aspects of life. As pointed out in chapter 7, the objectivization of these ideas in chemical morphology required detailed physiological, histological, and histochemical studies of the central and autonomic nervous systems, beginning with the *cell theory* of *Schleiden and Schwann* about 1840, and culminating in studies of the localization of cerebral sensory and motor functions in the human brain (*Penfield and Roberts,* 1955). These studies confirm *Peirce*'s (1891) analysis of the problem. From the philosophical point of view, the mind-body problem of *Descartes* can be approached from a position of *objective idealsm,* or the experimental method. The idea of performing experiments on the cortical centers required the experimental investigations of neurology carried out by investigators since the pioneering work of *von Helmholtz* in 1842 and *Kolliker* in 1846. Perception and knowledge in this and related fields of science required the organized efforts of hundreds of investigators. But these efforts necessarily presuppose the object of the search: the necessary condition of the psychic and physical factors in the structure and behavior of the human body and mind. The intense and continuous study of any definite scientific discipline must then be regarded as a special branch of anthropology.

Peirce's views as to the relation of scientific law to the principle of causality may be expressed by his explanation of the relationship between mechanical force and motion (*Joseph,* 1971a, b). When the law of motion is expressed as:

force = mass × acceleration,

the causal relationship between force and motion gives rise to a dualistic view in which many writers have felt compelled to accept force as an undefined idea. In statistical thermodynamics, it is necessary to clarify the relationships between causality, probability, and force functions in systems that are composed of many elementary units.

Difficulties in mechanics may often be resolved by stating the above equation in the form: 'force *is* the acceleration'. This is immediately recognized as one of *Newton*'s laws of motion. Thus, when the *law* is known, the idea of causality is replaced by a law of *necessity.* In this case again, '*Occam*'s razor' is applicable: a dualistic principle of cause and effect is replaced by a coherent unifying principle *of synechism* (chapter 13). This is a property of being organized or held together. It is also a principle of continuity and permanence. It applies to heterogeneous as well as to homogeneous physicochemical and biological systems.

It also applies to a necessary continuity between morphology and behavior. The relationship between the psychic and physical aspects of Cartesian dualism cannot be isolated one from the other, as in monism or neutralism. Thus, neither is an *absolute*, and the necessary connection is a *synechism*, which unifies all well-ordered purposeful biological events or *processes* (*Whitehead*, 1929). To attempt to isolate and identify each step in such a process is to enter a *labyrinth*, in which the principle of sufficient reason is required. This substitutes causality for law in a system of mechanistic materialism. Thus, the psychic aspects of Cartesian dualism are subordinated to the physical aspects, which are necessarily materialistic.

Monism, Dualism, and Pluralism

Two related sets of essays by *William James* were published in 1943 under the titles *Radical Empiricism* and *A Pluralistic Universe*. The former set (R.E.) was originally published in 1912, the latter (A.P.U.) in 1909. According to the editor, *Ralph Barton Perry*, these two sets represent 'the most important of *James'* metaphysical writings'.

In one of these essays, *Bergson and the Critique of Intellectualism*, it was shown that dynamic concepts become unintelligible when they are reduced to static concepts. According to *James*, a mathematical mind puts *motion* into a logical definition; it is conceived as 'the occupancy of serially successive points of space at serially successive instants of time'. This definition appears to sacrifice the sense-reality of the direct experience of motion to the intellectual vice of reductionism. In this case, an observable sense-experience involving a real synechistic *continuum* is reduced to an infinite series of discrete point-to-point correspondences that are conceived statically. This requires the arbitrary *intellectual* fallacy of analyzing an experienced process into its components, conceived to be isolable. According to *James*, this is a reductionist fallacy that is characteristic of a certain kind of rationalism. It is one of the aims of *James' Radical Empiricism* to avoid the type of absolutism characterized by intellectual abstractions, such as 'absolute' time and space.

Concepts are, of course, necessary to serve the practical purpose of organizing sense-data and experience for practical or 'pragmatic' purposes. This is likewise *Peirce*'s idea of the main function of any scientific conceptual scheme. Rather than in 'monism' or 'neutralism', this requires the problem of Cartesian dualism to imply the third method of treatment, i.e. 'objective idealism'. This presupposes the organization of the primary sense-data into scientific data assembled for the most practical purposes. Science must deal with irreducible processes and events rather than with isolable static entities.

A given process or event in biology always involves many sets and subsets of morphological and metabolic entities and processes. Unless the process can be expressed as a general law, it necessarily involves a continuum that can be expressed only as an infinite series of point-to-point biunivocal correspondences between primary morphological and secondary behavioral processes. The reality is inscrutable until the general laws of physicochemical and behavioral correspondences are revealed. According to the views of *Peirce* and of *James,* this requires the metaphysics of objective idealism or radical empiricism rather than any purely intellectual system of *a priori* rationalism.

In his *Essays on Radical Empiricism, James* everywhere emphasizes the abstract nature of all forms of rationalism, as contrasted with the concreteness of everyday human existence and experience. Rationalism in philosophy leads to ideas of the absolute: this attributes reality to transcendental ideas. 19th century forms of idealism, especially strong in Germany, are unscientific, and 'non-operational', however comforting the existence of various forms of absolute perfectionism may be to certain natures.

James considers such kinds of transcendental idealism or rationalism to yield a 'pragmatic' philosophy, in which concepts and percepts are practically enriched by the enlargement of concrete human experience of all kinds. This is a philosophy of *'thickness',* as contrasted with the *'thinness'* of non-empirical forms of rationalism. These views are expounded not only in *Essays in Radical Empiricism* and *A Pluralistic Universe,* but also in *Pragmatism* (1908).

To illustrate his point, *James* singled out as an example the little known figure of *Gustav Theodor Fechner* (1803—1887). During his long life in Leipzig, *Fechner* was actively engaged in many fields of scientific endeavor. He is well remembered for original researches in psychophysiology, including the well-known law of *Weber-Fechner.* This established a quantitative law relating sensory responses to the intensity of stimulation. 'It is the intense concreteness of *Fechner,* his fertility of detail, which fills me with (an) admiration ...' (*James,* 1909).

Fechner's experience in science was especially fecund. Although he was a qualified doctor of medicine, he spent his life as a professor of physics. His publications included extensive treatises in both physics and chemistry. His own publications in these fields were numerous and extensive. His original work included studies in galvanism, optics, and atomic theory. He is regarded by many as one of the most important founders of experimental psychology, as well as parapsychology. Thus, he exemplifies to an extreme the paradigmatic model of a philosopher whose experience is concrete and *thick,* as compared with the *thinness* of philosophies characterized by monistic idealism.

This emphasis on the richness (or thickness) of concrete experience coincides with *James'* philosophy of radical empiricism, based largely on his experience as a pioneer in psychology. Everywhere *James* expresses his disdain for *absolutist* or *monistic* concepts in idealist thought, which he characterizes as *thin* and purely intellectualist in nature. Hence, *James'* thought is pluralistic, concrete, and directed toward purposeful results in the world of human experience. In this, it is allied with the philosophies of his contemporaries, *Peirce* and *Bergson,* as well as with the thought of many later psychologists and philosophers, who emphasize the richness and thickness of human experience as pluralistic 'gestalten'.

Neuromuscular Irritability

The pragmatist philosophers, *Peirce, James,* and their followers, would probably agree with *Schopenhauer* in placing voluntarism, or *will* and *volition* at least on a par with *idea* as the basis of human conceptions of the world. Both will and idea originate in human or animal experience in a multidimensional pluralistic universe. Any attempt to reduce human thought and behavior to a unidimensional scheme is a step away from a thick toward a thin conception of life. Overspecialization or extreme reductionism in any branch of science might possibly increase knowledge of some isolated aspect of existence or essence, but this would likely result in the thinness of a narrowed abstraction.

As pointed out in the preceding chapter, abstractions of any kind originate in the neural sensations that are transmitted to sensory centers in the cerebral cortex. Stimuli originating from energy sources in the external world activate sensory nerve endings of various kinds. The transmitted impulses are conveyed by afferent fibers in the cerebral cortex, and are essential in the functions of perception and understanding.

The external sense impressions are necessary but not entirely sufficient sources of human ideas. The cortical sensory centers also receive impressions from internal afferent fibers and proprioceptors in the central and autonomic systems. These afferent fibers connect various parts of the brain with all other parts of the periphery and with the internal viscera. Thus, the conceptual world of perceptions and ideas is multidimensional and *thick* rather than monistic and *thin,* as in the schemes of absolutist philosphers or of reductionist scientists.

Thus, the world of 'will and idea' is internal as well as external. It is animal in nature, rather than transcendental. Thus, it is conceivable only in relation to the animal protoplasmic responses in the neuromuscular systems of real animals and of man. The concept of protoplasmic voluntarism necessarily implies the related concepts of purposeful organization and of goal-directed behavior in a pluralistic universe. This is multi-dimensional and irreducible to idealist abstractions.

As pointed out in chapter 7, the cell theory of *Schleiden and Schwann* dates from about the same period as the concept of protoplasm (*Purkinje,* 1825). Early studies of the histology of the nervous system include those of *von Helmholtz* of 1842 and *Kolliker* of 1846. The 19th century witnessed a continuous development of studies on the structure and behavior of the vertebrate and invertebrate nervous systems, including brain and sense organs (*Parker,* 1918).

Almost 2 centuries earlier than the work of *Schleiden and Schwann,* definite ideas as to the irritability of various organs and of skeletal muscle had been advanced (*Glisson,* 1650; *von Haller,* 1753; *Foster,* 1970). At about the same time as *Glisson*'s work, ideas as to the state of intramuscular water were advanced by *Stensen* (1664). Intracellular water was not regarded as homogeneous or perfectly mixed; it was considered to be structured and heterogeneous, consisting of coexistent states (intrafibrillar, interfibrillar, and membranous). These were not to be regarded as inert, but rather to be regarded as highly reactive, changing state with the physiological behavior of the muscle (*Joseph,* 1973).

In 1892, *Peirce* published an essay entitled *Man's Glassy Essence,* in which he described the organization, reactivity, and physicochemical state of protoplasm (life slimes) in various states of aggregation in such various organisms as the ameba, the slime mold, and in mammalian skeletal muscle. The typical state of protoplasm in any type of cell is solid or nearly solid in the resting state, and liquid or nearly liquid in the stimulated or active state. Thus, reactivity implies a change of biological water from one state of aggregation to the other.

According to *Peirce,* 'The liquefaction of protoplasm is accompanied by a mechanical phenomenon. Namely some kinds exhibit a tendency to draw themselves up into a globular form. This happens particularly with the contents of muscle cells. The prevalent opinion, founded on some of the most exquisite experimental investigations that the history of science can show, is undoubtedly that the contraction of muscle cells is due to osmotic pressure; it must be allowed that is a factor in producing the effect.'

Now osmotic pressure in physical chemistry or thermodynamics is one of four 'colligative properties' related to the chemical potential of each of the five physiological ions (Na, K, Ca, Mg, and Cl). For example, in the case of sodium:

$$\Delta\mu_{Na} = \Delta\mu^{\circ} + RT \ln \frac{c_{Na}{''}}{c_{Na}{'}},$$

where $\Delta\mu_{Na}$ is the change of chemical potential, and $\Delta\mu_{Na}{}^{\circ}$ is the change of standard chemical potential of the sodium ion. The value of $\Delta\mu_{Na}{}^{\circ}$ in any intracellular change of water is given by:

$$\Delta\mu_{Na}{}^{\circ} = \frac{164}{b_{Na}}\left(\frac{1}{D''} - \frac{1}{80}\right).$$

This is related to the electrostatic energy of hydration (*Born,* 1920; *Laidler and Pegis,* 1957).

The change of state of water is determined by the change of dielectric constant of water from the intramuscular value D'' to the value in pure liquid water of 80. As shown in chapter 3, the value of the free energy or maximal work of contraction is determined from the dielectric energy, $c_{Na}'' \Delta\mu_{Na}°$. The change of standard chemical potential can be determined from the action potential by a simple conversion:

$$E_a = 43.4 \, \Delta\mu_{Na}°,$$

where the action potential, E_a, is measured in millivolts and $\Delta\mu_{Na}°$ is estimated in kcal. An action potential of 120 mV thus corresponds to a change of standard chemical potential of about 2.8 kcal (*Joseph*, 1973). When required, the value of b_{Na}, the 'corrected' radius of the sodium ion, is taken as 1.25 Å units (*Laidler and Pegis*, 1957). Since the normal intracellular concentration of sodium, c_{Na}'', is about 0.028 mole/kg water, the value of the dielectric energy is given by:

$$c_{Na}'' \, \Delta\mu° = 0.028 \times 2.8 = 78.4 \text{ cal}$$
$$= 330 \text{ J/kg water.}$$

This agrees well with observed figures in various kinds of human skeletal muscle (*Joseph*, 1973; *Catchpole and Joseph*, 1974). Thus, as *Peirce* reasoned in *Man's Glassy Essence*, muscular contraction is related to a change of state of water, electrolytes, and protoplasm. This is accompanied by changes of all the properties that are related to the intracellular state of water. Muscle contraction and work can be understood only on the basis of the thermodynamics of heterogeneous systems (*Joseph*, 1971a, b; *Catchpole and Joseph*, 1974). An additional relation between dielectric energy and tension can also be derived (chapter 3). This can also be calculated from $c_{Na}'' \, \Delta\mu_{Na}°$. A value of 3,020 g/cm^2 is yielded for the maximal isometric tension. This also involves a change of state of water corresponding to a resting value of 30 for D'' to a value of 80 in the stimulated state. In all such changes of state, the following parameters are altered: metabolic rates, type of metabolism, maximal work and tension, and all other properties related to osmotic pressure and the chemical potentials of soluble components, including electrolytes, metabolites, and activated complexes (*Joseph*, 1973). Since the contraction involves only one degree of freedom, all the secondary properties of the muscle fibers are coordinated with one independent variable: the change of state of aggregation of protoplasm.

Auditory Reception and Transmission

It should be evident from many common observations that the auditory nerve endings of man are very sensitive to sound waves of very low intensity and of relatively high frequencies. For example, musical tones corresponding to frequencies of 200–300 vibrations/sec are not far from the note of 'middle C' on the piano keyboard. Pitches in this range correspond approximately to the frequency of vibration of the wings of a small insect such as a bee or a housefly. The intensity of the sound would at most correspond to the dielectric energy of the muscular contractions in the insect wing.

Normal basal metabolism is of the order of 2,000 kcal/day for a man who weighs 70 kg. The weight of a bee is about 70 mg, or about one millionth the weight of a man. The basal metabolism of mammals or of insects is proportional to the surface area, rather than to the weight. It is easily shown that surface area decreases by a factor of ten for each 1,000-fold decrease of weight. According to the 'principle of similitude', basal metabolism tends to be proportional to the two thirds power of the weight (*Thompson,* 1944). Applying this principle, the basal metabolism of an insect (70 mg) would be 20 kcal/day, as compared with the value of 2,000 kcal/day for a man of 70 kg. Thus, a bee that weighs 70 mg would produce about 1 kcal of metabolic energy per hour. This amounts to about 2.8×10^{-4} kcal/min, or about 5×10^{-6} kcal/sec (5×10^{-3} gcal). Let us assume that 20% of this energy is converted to audible sound waves resulting from the motion of the wings during flight. This amounts to 10^{-3} gcal/sec. Energy of this magnitude is thus sufficient to excite the nerve endings of the human auditory nerve.

The total number of neurones in the human brain is of the order of 10 billion. The dielectric energy of the brain may be estimated as 50 cal or 5×10^{-9} gcal/neurone. Dielectric energy of this order of magnitude may be thought to be available in the receptor endings of the auditory nerve. The sensitivity of each ending would thus correspond to sound intensity of the order of 10^{-6} to 10^{-5} gcal/sec, depending on the total number of endings exposed to the oscillatory wave energy. This is sufficient to respond to the wing motion of a small insect. A sustained pitch or tone of this order of magnitude would correspond to the reception of about 100 gcal or 0.1 kcal/day, or about 20% of the basal metabolism, since it has been assumed that only that fraction of the dielectric energy of the wing motion is transmitted to the nerve endings.

It is evident from this that emission and perception of audible sound waves are processes that depend on high frequency vibrations of the protoplasm in both the sensory endings of the auditory nerve, as well as in the protoplasm where the sound waves originate. In the above example, the sound waves originated as oscillatory dielectric energy of the wing muscles. In human speech and communication, the sound waves originate as oscillatory vibrations in the vocal cords of the speaker. The tension of these muscles can be voluntarily controlled in the speech centers of the cortex; it determines the pitch or frequency of the sound waves. Intensity is determined by the rate of emission of air from the lungs through the windpipe and vocal cords. The quality of the sound also depends on voluntary muscular control of the oral cavity, throat, tongue, and lips.

The normal basal metabolism of man is about 80 kcal/h. In conversation, the level may be elevated by about 50%, or 40 kcal/h. If the transmission of energy through the auditory nerve endings to the brain centers occurs at the rate of 5×10^{-9} kcal/sec/auditor, this amounts to about 2×10^{-4} kcal/h. Thus, 40 kcal/h is a rate of energy production that is sufficient to provide threshold audibility to 2,000 auditors. However, only a fraction of the sound energy would reach the nerve endings. This depends on many acoustical factors, indluding reasonance of the room or auditorium and absorption of a fraction of the sound. Therefore, the figure of 2,000 auditors would represent a maximal number. The actual number might be of the order of 100—500, for example. The above example, however, sufficiently indicates the principle that 40 kcal of vocal energy per hour is sufficient to activate resonant protoplasmic oscillations in the nerve endings of a large number of auditors under favorable conditions. Thus, vocal communication implies voluntary transmission originating in oscillatory changes of state of protoplasmic water in the respiratory and vocal passages of the speaker, terminating in resonant oscillations in the neuroplasm of the auditor. All such communication depends on very delicate responses of protoplasm to voluntary controls in both sets of muscular and sensory (afferent) and effector (efferent) fibers. The brain behaves as a 'relay' in coordinating afferent sensations and perceptions with voluntary responses.

Chapter 9

Organicism

Above certain levels in the phylogenetic scale of vertebrates in the animal kingdom, there is a necessary principle of order or invariance that permits classification of species into various classes and orders that distinguish warm-blooded from cold-blooded vertebrates. Many kinds of classification and sub-classification of animals have long been recognized by biologists. These have to do with anatomical structure, with phylogeny and ontogeny, with environmental adaptations, mating, and sexual habits and behavior, and with many other vital phenomena.

Survival of any mammalian species over long periods of time requires selective adaptations to a terrestrial or marine environment, which has the property of 'fitness'. Most mammalian species are terrestrial, and are character-ized by locomotion in a horizontal position. Others like squirrels and chipmunks are adapted to vertical or climbing types of locomotion, and are able to execute rather intrepid leaps. Animals in general and quadrupeds, in particular, can be recognized by their characteristic gaits; because of the great number and variety of these types of locomotion, it is unnecessary to labor this matter in detail. It is only necessary to point out that animal locomotion depends on anatomy. Locomotion is thus an *emergent* property that cannot be reduced to its com-ponent muscles, myofibrils, joints, nervous reflex arcs, and cerebral centers in any sense of *isolation*. The concept of organism is necessarily integrative. Any special form of locomotion, walking, running, climbing, swimming, or crawling, depends on the nature of the external environment. The human body is adapted either to climbing or descending a given staircase, ladder, or hill. In such an act, the motion is organized by sensory and motor centers in the cerebral cortex, which respond to afferent stimuli from all the sense organs and to proprioceptive messages from the peripheral neuromuscular system. Such acts of climbing or descending are highly integrated and purposeful, and involve both will and idea (chapter 7).

Thus, the concept of organism necessarily involves reciprocal states of order or disorder in all the related anatomical structures, brain centers, and sense organs. The responses are purposeful, goal-directed, and well-ordered in the normal organism. Since they are always related to changes in the brain, sense organs, and neuromuscular system, they imply corresponding changes in the

chemical morphology and respiratory metabolism in all the anatomical structures. These imply changes of configurational entropy and free energy in active
protoplasm related to work, tension, and nerve impulses. According to the
results of chapter 3 (*Carnot*'s principle) and chapter 7 (voluntarism), such
physiological responses imply changes in the free energy of hydration, and in
other dielectric properties of intracellular phases.

Changes of respiratory metabolism, such as oxygen consumption, production of heat, and carbon dioxide, are likewise responsive to labile changes of
state of intracellular water. Thus, all the mechanical, electrical, and metabolic
processes are correlated with hydration energy and the standard chemical
potentials of the physiological ions (*Joseph,* 1973; *Catchpole and Joseph,* 1974).

A high coordination of all behavioral processes with internal changes in the
anatomical, morphological, and physicochemical systems are characteristic of
living organisms; they are inconceivable in *mechanisms,* which rely on movements of non-protoplasmic masses. In *Peirce*'s essay, *Man's Glassy Essence,* he
considers the lability of intramuscular protoplasm to depend on the intracellular
changes of state of water. Thus, intracellular water may be observed to serve
several distinct physiological or biological functions. These include an energy
providing function in its change of state from a well-ordered solid condition to a
disordered semi-liquid state of high dielectric constant. In this state, it changes
its character from a non-polar to a polar solvent for carbohydrates, amino acids,
phosphate esters, and inorganic electrolytes. A change in the solvent properties
implies simultaneous changes in the tension or length of muscle fibers and in
changes of the electrical properties (action potentials and nerve conduction).
Thus, the following sets of properties are coordinated with intracellular changes
of water: (1) muscular tension and work; (2) electrical properties such as action
potentials, and (3) mechanical properties related to dielectric energy and hydration energy, as measured by the change of standard chemical potential, $\Delta\mu_{Na}°$.

These groups of properties are well-ordered and highly coordinated with
changes of state of the labile intracellular water. Thus, cells and tissues are
continually changing intracellular and extracellular states of water inseparably
from changes in measurable secondary properties: mechanical, electrical, and
metabolic. These are *emergent* properties which are integrated and organismic
only in the normal intact animal.

Since in the normally functioning animal or human organism, will and idea
are held together by a principle of 'synechism' (chapter 13), the principle of
Occam's razor (chapter 8) can be applied to unify the entire organism, as an
emergent of all its cells and tissues (*Wheeler,* 1928; *Joseph,* 1973). Then it would
be unnecessary to apply *James'* principle of 'pluralism' to coordinate all the
separate parts, which are normally inseparable.

In *The Creative Mind* (1946), *Bergson* has included an essay on *The
Philosophy of Claude Bernard,* in which he discusses some of the main problems

of the experimental method in physiology, the relation of that science to physics and chemistry, and the distinguishing features of the organicist point of view, as discussed in *An Introduction to the Study of Experimental Medicine* (*Bernard*, 1878). It is evident according to *Bergson* that *Bernard* everywhere attacks those who refuse to acknowledge physiology as a special or independent science distinct from physics and chemistry. Although physicochemical phenomena are everywhere evident, there is always in biology or in 'vital phenomena' something that cannot be *reduced* to the atomic or molecular level. 'He is not a physiologist who has not the organizing sense of that special coordination of the parts to the whole, characteristic of the vital phenomenon. In the living being things take place as though a certain "idea" stepped in, which took into account the order in which the elements are grouped' (*Bergson*, 1946, p. 205).

In taking into account this principle of 'order', we have a connecting link or bridge between *Bernard*'s concept of an organizing idea, and the thermodynamic concept of 'entropy' or 'negative entropy', as applied by *Boltzmann* (1905) and by *Schrodinger* (1944). Stability, order, and well-ordered morphology are also implicit in the application of the principle of *Carnot-Clausius* and *Gibbs'* phase rule to vital phenomena (*Joseph*, 1973). Physicochemical state and behavior then depend on the properties of the macromolecular aggregates of protoplasm and the life slimes (*Peirce*, 1878, 1892).

Order and 'negative entropy' are also implicit in the views of *Frey-Wyssling*, as applied to the purposeful behavior of submicroscopic protoplasmic morphology. Although the elementary physicochemical properties of non-living substances, such as water and the inorganic electrolytes, are inherent in vital phenomena, their behavior is never independent of the properties of protoplasm. Thus, a physiologist must see the 'organizing sense' of the *whole,* which includes the presence of the inorganic elements and water. According to *Macallum* (1910), the inorganic composition of the body must be regarded as an 'heirloom', surviving from the primitive cosmic environment (sea water) in which life and protoplasm may be conceived to have originated. The organicist 'idea' or 'will' cannot be conceived to be possible without taking into account the order in which the elements are grouped. The abstract organicist concept of 'order' attains concreteness by application of the principles of *Carnot* and of *Gibbs* (chapter 3).

Machines seem to be distinguishable from organisms by the fact that they are not designed to operate on sources of dielectric energy of hydration. As in living animals this would require an ultimate source of 'negative entropy' or 'configurational free energy' to maintain neuromuscular tone and irritability (*Boltzmann,* 1905; *Schrodinger,* 1944). In nature, the permanent source of 'negative entropy' is found in sunlight, as it acts on the process of photosynthesis in the green leaves of plants. Until man is able to produce colloidal systems of macromolecules, water, and electrolytes, it would seem that no machine that imitates the properties of irritable protoplasm could be constructed out of inorganic substances. At best, the human being seems limited to 'artificial brains', to mechanical computers, or to automatic 'robots', which are lacking in the true 'organizing sense' that is characteristic of protoplasmic organisms. According to *Bernard,* the physicist or engineer on whom we rely for the construction of robots or other automata is lacking in this organizing sense of the true physiologist, or student of the phenomena of life.

The Universe of Discourse

All species of multicellular animals or metazoa may be described by a certain number of essential properties which distinguishes a given species from any other. Thus, it has been shown (*Joseph,* 1973) that any living member of a species in the resting adult state is characterized by: (I) an invariant state of chemical morphology (M); (II) an invariant rate of basal metabolism, m, and (III) an invariant heterogeneous structure, H.

When I, II, and III are in the normal adult standard resting state, the actual living state corresponds to a state IV, which describes the 'universe of discourse' of logical relationships. A diagram of three equal circles of radius r can be drawn, in which the three centers describe an equilateral triangle; each side of which is of the length 2r, or d, the distance between any two centers. The three circles then intersect to form the area IV, which has the three following properties common to each member of the living species: (1) invariant heterogeneous morphology; (2) invariant basal metabolism, and (3) invariant heterogeneous structure. Thus, all living species are structured and heterogeneous.

This is the necessary condition for invariant chemical morphology and for constant respiratory metabolism of all cells and tissues. If such a system in the standard state can undergo any given change of state in the neuromuscular system this involves a change of chemical morphology of that part of the system. This is a *behavioral process,* which can be symbolized as P (for process). Then in the standard state, we have:

$$P \supset (M, m) \text{ (resting)},$$

and

$$P' \supset (M', m') \text{ (behavioral process)}.$$

Thus, in a behavioral process:

$$P (M, m) \supset P' (M', m'),$$

where M' is an altered state of chemical morphology in any structure or substructure, and m' is the corresponding altered metabolic state. The behavioral

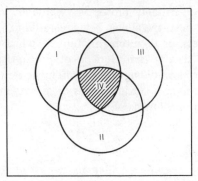

Fig. 1. Physicochemical conditions for invariance and reactivity of biological systems. I = set of all invariant systems; II = set of all reactive systems; III = set of all heterogeneous systems; IV = set of all systems that are invariant, heterogeneous, and reactive. All living cells and tissues are in set IV.

process also involes changes in all secondary functions that depend on M'. These may all be considered to depend on changes of dielectric constant, hydration energies, and altered chemical potentials of the ions. Changes of the solubilities of nutrients and metabolites likewise are related to the dielectric properties of water in differing states of aggregation.

These relationships are illustrated in figure 1, in which circle I represents the normal or modified state of chemical morphology, II represents the normal or altered state of respiratory metabolism, and III represents the normal or altered state behavioral state. The 'universe of discourse', IV, thus is described by concomitant changes of morphology, metabolism, and heterogeneous structure, as related to behavior. Thus, all neuromuscular processes of behavior and physiochemical state are ordered and unified by the underlying changes of dielectric constant, dielectric energy, and hydration energy of protoplasm between any two states of aggregation in each type of structure. Irritability and responses such as contractility, tension, and transmission all depend on the possible states of water throughout the system (*Joseph,* 1973). *Claude Bernard's* 'organizing sense of the whole' can be seen to be inherent in the 'universe of discourse' characteristic of all living organisms. This is the tendency of heterogeneous systems of protoplasm to be organized or to reorganize themselves by responses in which morphology, metabolism, and behavior are always unified, integrated, and coordinated by univariant processes, involving only one degree of freedom. The biological system remains univariant because of the operation of *Gibbs'* phase rule which operates to maintain all the constraining conditions that characterize the biological 'universe of discourse'. In this way, *Bernard's* organizing sense of the whole becomes related to *Carnot's* principle and *Gibbs'* 'equilibrium of heterogeneous substances'. Metabolizing cells and tissues must then conform to the same conditions of constraint that apply to all other systems of heterogeneous substances. The phase rule thus supplies the organizing sense characteristic of all such systems. In living organisms, the responses of protoplasm are always constrained by the existence of intracellular water in two or more labile states of aggregation. This affords a supply of configurational free energy or negative entropy related to the dielectric properties of the protoplasmic structures.

Monism and Dualism in Organism and Environment

From the foregoing considerations, it is evident that purposeful processes of biological behavior require well-ordered responses of protoplasmic structures and intracellular metabolic reactions in all cells and tissues of the body. From the point of view of physical chemistry, the responses involve coordinated changes of state of water in each kind of structure. Thus, each cell operates with one degree of freedom. This can be symbolized as:

$$A, B, C \ldots \supset X, Y, Z \ldots$$

where A, B, C ... represent a set of primary properties describing the intracellular standard state of water, electrolytes, and macromolecules. The symbol $\supset$ is read as 'implies'. Thus, the primary parameters of composition, structure, state, and temperature imply a set of secondary parameters (X, Y, Z ...). These refer to the chemical potentials of all components, chemical reactivities, and all dielectric properties, such as standard chemical potentials, hydration energies, and ion concentrations. Then in an excited or stimulated state,

$$A', B', C' \ldots X', Y', Z' \ldots$$

Here (X', Y', Z' ...) behaves as a univariant set. The response occurs with one degree of freedom with respect to any change of (A, B, C ...). Thus, a change of any of the parameters A, B, C ... in such a process as aging, growth, or development, for example, produces a well-ordered *unified* response in the set (X, Y, Z ...), corresponding to the secondary properties of the structure.

An example would be the change of state of heart muscle from systole to diastole in the normal heart. This occurs between two well-ordered states, in which:

$$S \rightarrow S'$$
Diastole   Systole

or

$$(X, Y, Z \ldots) \rightarrow (X', Y', Z' \ldots).$$

Here, the cardiac muscle contracts with one degree of freedom. All the secondary properties depend on one independent variable, which may be taken as the dielectric constant, the dielectric energy, the standard chemical potential of sodium, or the hydration energy. Thus, a change from one limiting state to a second state is a uni-dimensional process with one degree of freedom.

When the response of any kind of intracellular phase to any kind of stimulus is a well-ordered change between two well-ordered states of protoplasm, this usually implies that the phase is univariant. It is then necessary to inquire as to the nature of the independent variable or *argument*.

Components and Phases

The physicochemical state of any heterogeneous system is defined by the chemical composition of each phase, and by the external variables such as temperature, pressure, gravitational and electrical fields, and so forth. In biological systems at constant temperature and pressure, it is possible to treat all the external factors as constants, and to consider only composition and state as the significant parameters.

In very slow processes, such as growth, development, and aging of the body as a whole, all functions depend only on time. A variable is defined as a quantitiy that changes. If all possible changes occur only in time, then only time-dependent quantities need be treated as variables (*Frege,* 1952; *Joseph,* 1973). There are only small changes in the electrolyte-water composition of the *milieu intérieur* during the life span of human beings and other mammalian organisms (*Widdowson and Dickerson,* 1964). Therefore, blood plasma and other extracellular fluids can be treated as invariant in the normal resting state. Intracellular protoplasmic phases may show very considerable changes of water-electrolyte composition during processes of growth, development, and aging. All such functions of time must be treated as variables. In a univariant system, it is necessary to define the independent variable or *argument* that is the primary time-dependent magnitude. For this it is required to define the physicochemical system with respect to phases and components, considering the conditions of temperature and pressure to be fixed in the mammalian organism.

Two kinds of intracellular or protoplasmic constituents are considered. The primary time-dependent quantity is the macromolecular composition: proteins, lipids, carbohydrates, nucleic acids, and other substances of high molecular weight, which determine the physicochemical state at any time in the presence of an invariant *milieu intérieur*. It may be assumed at any time that the neuromuscular composition is described by n protoplasmic substances which may be regarded as *fixed* and immobile. The entire composition then depends on $(n + 6)$ intracellular substances, where the number 6 refers to water and the five inorganic ions: sodium, potassium, calcium, magnesium, and chloride. These inorganic ions are of extracellular origin, occurring in all body fluids, and in the external cosmic environment of all animals and plants. Thus, water and the electrolytes of primitive sea water are constituents of environmental origin, that are common to all protoplasmic structures. The n macromolecule substances of protoplasm are products of internal endogenous metabolism. They depend on the phylogeny and ontogeny of any species and are characteristic of each given kind of protoplasm. Thus, the primary time-dependent variable or argument in any given case is the protoplasmic composition as referred to the n macromolecular substances.

It is now necessary to consider the conditions for a resting state of protoplasm with one degree of freedom with respect to a standard growth curve for the organism. At any point on the growth curve, n may be treated as a constant at a given state of growth, age, and development. Then the composition of a given kind of intracellular phase must satisfy the following conditions of balance.

I. Constant chemical potentials of binary and ternary electrolytes:

$$\mu_{NaCl}' = \mu_{NaCl}'' \text{ (NaCl or KCl)},$$

where μ' refers to blood plasma, and μ'' refers to any other phase in a system of p phases (including plasma).

II. Constant chemical potential of water:

$$\mu_{H_2O}' = \mu_{H_2O}''$$

(in a system of p phases including blood plasma).

Conditions I and II establish water and electrolyte balance in all cells, tissues, and extracellular fluids of the *milieu intérieur*. For the five inorganic ions, these conditions imply additional constraints and restrictions of the form:

$$\Delta\mu_{Na} = \Delta\mu_K = \frac{1}{2}\Delta\mu_{Ca} = \frac{1}{2}\Delta\mu_{Mg} = -\Delta\mu_{Cl} = \delta. \tag{7}$$

In equation 7, δ is the equivalent change of chemical potential of each kind of ion (chapter III). For any kind of ion of this class (reversible transport):

$$\Delta\mu_i = \Delta\mu_i^\circ + RT \ln \frac{(c_i)''}{(c_i)'},$$

where $(c_i)''$ refers to the total intracellular concentration of the ith kind of ion (free plus bound). Here $\Delta\mu_i$ and $\Delta\mu_i^\circ$ refer respectively to the change of chemical potential and the change of standard chemical potential for the given kind of ion.

If, for simplicity, the state is referred only to the three univalent ions (Na,

K, and Cl), three parameters for each kind of ion must be considered: $\Delta\mu_i$, $\Delta\mu_i^\circ$, and $(c_i)''$. Thus, to describe the intracellular state of these kinds of ion, a total of nine parameters must be considered. This requires a total of nine equations for any invariant point on the resting growth curve. According to the foregoing, the necessary conditions include the following:

(a) $\Delta\mu_{Na} = \Delta\mu_K = -\Delta\mu_{Cl}$ (two equations),

(b) $\Delta\mu_i^\circ = f(D'')$ (three equations, one for each kind of ion),

(c) $\Delta\mu_i = \Delta\mu_i^\circ + RT \ln \dfrac{(c_i)''}{(c_i)'}$,

where $(c_i)'$ is constant for each kind of ion. Thus, a, b, and c supply a total of nine equations required to determine the three parameters for each of the three kinds of ion. However, it has been necessary to introduce two arbitrary parameters: D'', the intracellular dielectric constant, and x, the colloidal charge. Each of these parameters depends on the intracellular composition with respect to the n macromolecular substances. Thus, generally speaking, D'' and x cannot vary independently; each is a function of growth, age, and development. Thus, D'' and x form a conjugated set of properties that are determined by the primary set of n intracellular substances. Hence they imply the *ninth* condition for an invariant system at any point on the standard growth curve. This implies one degree of freedom when the curve is extended to include significant changes of composition and state. To summarize the necessary conditions for invariance, these include:

(1) Two equations relating $\Delta\mu_i$ for three kinds of ions. (2) Three equations relating $\Delta\mu_i^\circ$ to D''. (3) Three equations relating $\Delta\mu_i$ and $\Delta\mu_i^\circ$) to $(c_i)''$. (4) One equation relating $\Sigma(c_i)''$ to x, the colloidal charge.

The number of degrees of freedom, f, is defined as the number of independent conditions necessary to determine δ, the equivalent change of chemical potential of Na, K, and Cl ions. When the two arbitrary parameters, D'' and x, depend only on age, growth, and development, the system is univariant, and is determined by the intracellular composition of n fixed macromolecular substances. Thus, for the resting state of any given structure, intracellular protoplasm is univariant. This implies that the significant variables are related to chemical morphology and the intracellular state of water.

Muscular Behavior

Muscular contraction, as studied experimentally, is accompanied, among other things, by the following observable changes: (1) A rapid change of electromotive force, measured as the action potential, E_a. (2) An observable 'spike potential', E_{Na}, observed at the peak of the action potential. This measures the limit of a 'depolarization' phase of the process. (3) A recovery period of depolarization of a few milliseconds, after which the resting potential, E, is again observed. (4) A rapid phase of isotonic contraction, during which external work may be performed. (5) Production of heat in the recovery period (step 3). (6) Formation of lactic acid, inorganic phosphate, and free creatine during rapid anaerobic contraction. (7) Formation of CO_2 and uptake of oxygen during aerobic contraction.

Depending on the exact conditions of constraint in such experimental procedures, many side effects may be observed: these are related to physiological effects, such as changes of acid-base balance, water-electrolyte balance, and muscular fatigue. Recovery to the physiological standard state of homeostasis requires a set of favorable conditions in the extracellular milieu.

The uncontracted or 'relexed' state of the muscle fibers is therefore well-ordered (low entropy), as compared with the disordered state of contraction (high entropy). Thus, contraction involves a release of configurational free energy (or increase of entropy) related to the tension and length of the muscle fibers. Reversal of the process requires a supply of 'negative entropy' originating in intracellular supplies of glucose or glycogen (*Joseph,* 1973). Adenosine triphosphate (ATP) enters the process during the polarization rather than in the depolarization process, as commonly assumed (*Catchpole and Joseph,* 1974). Along with other organic phosphates, it enters into the anaerobic breakdown of glucose in several steps of conversion of carbohydrates to lactic acid. This process is necessary in the repolarization process to restore the fibers to the polarized state of high free energy and low configurational entropy. The glycolytic process is accelerated by the conversion of water to a polar solvent, differing from the resting state of low dielectric constant, in which it behaves as a non-polar solvent. This suppresses glycolysis and lowers the respiratory quotient.

In order to establish the physicochemical and thermodynamic basis for muscular contraction under either isotonic or isometric conditions, it is necessary again to consider the phase rule conditions for water-electrolyte balance, as well as the thermodynamic conditions for external work, for isometric tension, and for anaerobic glycolytic metabolism (*Joseph,* 1973).

The fundamental equation for reversible electromotive force in the standard resting state is obtained from *Gibbs'* equations 687 and 688:

$$FE + \delta = O,$$

where E is the electromotive force, F is the Faraday constant, and δ is the equivalent change of chemical potential of each of the five inorganic physiological ions: Na, K, Ca, Mg, and Cl. When E is expressed in volts, F may be taken either as 96,500 C/J, or as 23,060 C/cal. Then δ is expressed either as 43.4 mV/

kcal, or as 10.4 mV/J. A typical value of E for resting mammalian skeletal muscle may be taken as -80 mV. Then the value of $\delta \ \Delta\mu_{Na}$ is calculated as 1.84 kcal. This value depends on the change of standard chemical potential and on the ratio of c_{Na}'' to c_{Na}', (where this is expressed as r_{Na}). Thus:

$$\Delta\mu_{Na} = \Delta\mu_{Na}° + RT \ln r_{Na}.$$

A typical value of r_{Na} in mammalian skeletal muscle is 0.20, when c_{Na}'' is taken as 0.028 mole/kg water, and c_{Na}' is taken as 0.140 mole/kg.

At 37 °C, the expression converts to:

$$\Delta\mu_{Na} = \Delta\mu_{Na}° + 1.40 \log_{10} (0.20) \ (kcal),$$

or

$$\Delta\mu_{Na}° = 1.84 + 0.99 = 2.83 \ kcal.$$

This corresponds to an action potential of 123 mV. Thus:

$$E = E° + E_{Na}$$

or

$$-80 = -122.9 + 42.9 \ (mV).$$

The 'spike potential' is then given by:

$$E_{Na} = 61.3 \log_{10} r_{Na} = 61.3 \log_{10} (0.20) = 42.9 \ mV.$$

When, for convenience, $\Delta\mu_{Na}°$ is taken as 3 kcal, and $\Delta\mu_{Na}$ as 2 kcal, we have:

$$E = -86.8 \ mV; \ E_a = 130.2 \ mV, \ and \ E_{Na} = 43.4 \ mV.$$

These correspond fairly well with the average values for normal mammalian skeletal muscle. The change of standard chemical potential of sodium ion is estimated as about 2.8 kcal from the above figures. The dielectric energy, expressed as cal/kg water is then:

$$c_{Na}'' \ \Delta\mu_{Na}° = 0.028 \times 2.8 \times 1,000 = 78.4 \ cal$$

(*Catchpole and Joseph,* 1974). This converts to 334 kg/m/kg water. Since the water content of the human arm muscles (biceps and brachialis) is about 250 g, the calculated dielectric energy is approximately 334/4, or 83.5 ca/m. This is within 10% of the value of 9 kg/m for the maximal work of the arm muscles in athletic record performances (*Hill*, 1944; *Catchpole and Joseph*, 1974). This applies also to the muscles of the leg, as in the performance of the high jump or sprint (*Joseph*, 1971a, b). Thus, as a first approximation, the maximal work content is proportional to $c_{Na}'' \Delta\mu_{Na}^{\circ}$, the dielectric energy. Now according to chapter VII,

$$c_{Na}'' \Delta\mu_{Na}^{\circ} = 164 \left(\frac{1}{D''} - \frac{1}{80} \right),$$

where D'' is the resting intracellular dielectric constant, and 80 is the dielectric constant of liquid water. Dielectric energy of 9 kg/m corresponds to a value of about 30 for the uncontracted muscle. The maximal work of contraction is related to the free energy change, ΔG, by the formula:

$$\Delta G = -W = -78.4 \text{ cal.}$$

Also:

$$\Delta G = -T\Delta S = -78.4 \text{ cal.}$$

Therefore, contraction depends on a change of state involving an increase of configurational entropy, as well as an increase of dielectric constant.

Chapter 10

Growth of the Mind

In the 20th century, two major lines of development in the scientific study of human knowledge and behavior have tended to support the philosophical ideas of *Locke* and *Hume* insofar as they referred to the empirical or *a postiori* basis of human knowledge and behavior. The first of these developments has occurred in the field of child psychology and education. Major advances in these fields of study are associated with the work of *Piaget* which, beginning about 1920, has continued through several subsequent decades. These studies were concerned with the child's perception of space, time, and motion, and with his ability to communicate these perceptions through linguistic comprehension of the ideas of number, distance, duration, and elementary notions of logical classification. These mental functions continue well beyond the age of adolescence into maturity. Ideas, perceptions, knowledge, and beliefs are then structured to become the heritage of any human group or society.

Structured behavior is also characteristic of primitive or 'savage' human societies, as has been shown in many ways by the anthropological studies of *Levi-Strauss* (1970). Among the topics treated by *Levi-Strauss* are language and kinship, social organizations, the functions of symbolism, the structure of myths, and various forms of ritual. In one form or another, all these kinds of structure are common to all human societies, and enter into the very core of human behavior, beginning in infancy, and continuing through the periods of growth, adolescence, and maturity.

Growth and Development

At any age after birth, the human being of either sex is characterized by anatomical and morphological development, and by acquired knowledge, perceptions, abilities, and skills in all the permitted or required ranges of the inherited social or anthropological structures. The ability at any given age to exercise any given function depends on the growth and development of the neuromuscular system in all its parts — brain, especially the cerebral cortex, sense organs, including the auditory and motor speech centers, and the entire peripheral system of nerve and skeletal muscle. The combined and integrative action of the entire system is necessary to the full acquisition of the 'sense of organism' in everything related to the concepts of space, time, and number, as related to the full development of human cognition and understanding.

Thus, human knowledge and understanding are developed according to *a postiori* experience; the principles of *Locke* and *Hume* are thus confirmed by the experience of scientific disciplines. Experience has also tended to refute the idea of *Kant* that there are innate *a priori* ideas of space, time, and causality. These ideas are acquired early in infancy or childhood only as the result of experience. Difficult concepts related to number, quantity, and the logic of classes and aggregates are acquired with more difficulty. Often such difficulties persist into the human adult period. These concepts apply to well-organized mental operations of human beings; possibly they are completely inaccessible to other species.

In the following pages, water-electrolyte balance in the developing skeletal muscle in the fetal, postpartum and adult periods of human beings will be compared with figures for brain in the same periods of life. Similar data for muscle and brain will be shown for the pig. From the data, the following calculations may be made according to the principles of earlier chapters and of earlier publications (*Joseph,* 1971a, b; 1973). (1) Changes of standard chemical potential of sodium $\Delta\mu_{Na}°$, referred to blood plasma. (2) Dielectric energy, $c_{Na}"$ $\Delta\mu_{Na}°$. (3) Dielectric constant. (4) Mean equivalent weight of cellular colloid.

The data and calculations supply information regarding the rates of development of skeletal muscle and brain in the mammalian organism. Presumably, biological behavior in any species would depend on growth rates of the neuromuscular system. In the human being, knowledge, understanding, perception, will and idea, or in fact the entire learning process would necessarily be directed and constrained by measurable physicochemical parameters, as they develop from childhood to maturity.

The following calculations (table I) from the data of *Widdowson and Dickerson* (1964) may be compared with earlier estimates (*Joseph,* 1973). Among human tissues, skeletal muscle shows the greatest changes from the fetal to the adult state. As will be shown in the following pages, the changes in liver, heart, kidney, and brain are of similar orders of magnitude. This may be related to the fact that these four tissues are probably actively functioning in the later periods of fetal life, as well as in newborn and postpartum infants. Of all these tissues, skeletal muscle shows the greatest changes of dielectric properties during the postpartum growth period.

Similar calculations for the skeletal muscle of the growing rat are shown in table II (*Hazlewood and Nichols,* 1969; *Joseph,* 1973).

A comparison of tables I and II with respect to the development of rat and human skeletal muscle shows the following similarities. In the early fetal period of human beings (13–22 weeks), the dielectric constant, $D"$, is of the order of

60—64, as compared with values of 63—68 for rats of the age of 2—4 days. In the adult period, human muscle shows a value of 31 for D'', as compared to 28 found for the 65-day rat.

In the human being, dielectric energy ranges from 42.57 cal/kg water in the fetus to 80.60 cal/kg water in the adult, an increase of nearly 100%. Comparable values in the young rat are 41.54—46.50 cal/kg water (2—4 days), increasing to 80.84 or 79.99 cal at 32 or 65 days.

Thus, the range of variation in the growth period of human beings is quite similar to that found in growing rats. In each species, the increase of dielectric energy is of the order of 100% between the limits of high to low dielectric constant (about 65—30). This is correlated with a decrease of intracellular water from about 90% to a value of about 75—79% (*Joseph,* 1973).

Thus, the fundamental process in the growth and development of skeletal muscle is the synthesis of muscle proteins, which increase from a newborn level of about 10% to an adult level of the order of 25%. This increase is paralleled by an increase of the mean equivalent weight of the muscle colloids — 1,200—2,160 g/Eq (human) and 1,220—1,940 g/Eq (rat). Thus, there is a change in the relative properties of the intramuscular proteins as well as an increase in the total protein content. A value of 1,000 g/Eq in fetal muscle would correspond to a high level of phosphorus to nitrogen or of nucleic acids to total protein. In the adult state, the mean equivalent weight increases to a value of the order of 2,000 g/Eq — this corresponds to a decrease of the ratio of phosphorus to nitrogen, corresponding to an increase of the contractile proteins, actin, and myosin, as compared to the increase of nucleic acids. Thus, muscle develops primarily with respect to the nuclear components, which are mainly related to macromolecular synthesis and organization rather than to dielectric energy or total work capacity and isometric tension (*Joseph,* 1973).

Whereas there are many variables in the growing human or mammalian organism, there may be only a small number of *independent* variables, or degrees of freedom. Thus, if f denotes the number of degrees of freedom, v, the total number of variables, and u, the number of conditions of constraint:

$$f = v - u,$$

or

Degrees of freedom = total number of variables minus number of conditions of constraint.

This represents an expression of *Gibbs'* (1875, 1928) phase rule, as applied to biological systems (*Joseph,* 1971a, b; 1973). In a normal living organism, it would always be possible to say that the number of degrees of freedom, f, is always a relatively small number. This expresses the biological fact that living organisms belong to a class of well-ordered cohesive physicochemical systems. According to the results of tables I and II, it is evident that all the variables of developing muscle are related to protein synthesis, dielectric properties, and mean equivalent weight of the intracellular colloids. This is a result of the fact that all variations are functions of time, growth, and development.

Table I. Electrolyte balance in growth and development

	Fetus		New-born	4–7 months	Adult
	13–14 weeks	20–22 weeks			
Human skeletal muscle					
$c_{Na}''\,\Delta\mu_{Na}°$, cal	42.87	56.39	77.31	57.78	80.60
$\Delta\mu_{Na}°$, kcal	0.39	0.56	1.35	1.28	2.81
D''	64	60	43	45	31
Equiv. wt, g	1,200	1,210	2,200	1,500	2,160
Human brain					
$c_{Na}''\,\Delta\mu_{Na}°$, cal	46.93	46.59	53.51	47.90	
$\Delta\mu_{Na}°$, kcal	0.44	0.45	0.59	0.67	
D''	63	43	57	57	
Equiv. wt, g	1,050	980	1,200	1,710	
Distribution of dielectric energy					
Body weight, kg	0.31	2.53	2.73	70	
Dielectric energy, kcal/kg body weight[1]	137	22.6	28.3	1.14	
Dielectric energy, cal/kg body weight[2]	145	18.4	19.7	0.68	
Ratio (brain to skeletal muscle)	1.05	0.81	0.69	0.60	

[1] Skeletal muscle; [2] Brain.

Table II. Electrolyte balance in growth period of rats[1]

	Age, days					
	2	4	8	16	32	65
$c_{Na}''\,\Delta\mu_{Na}°$, cal	41.54	46.50	61.40	72.54	80.84	79.98
$\Delta\mu_{Na}°$, kcal	0.37	0.44	0.87	1.65	2.72	3.32
D''	68	63	52	40	30	28
Equiv. wt, g	1,090	1,220	1,540	1,830	1,850	1,940

[1] From Hazlewood and Nichols (1969) and Joseph (1973).

It is now necessary to ask the question 'What is a variable?' This is answered by the reply: 'A variable is a quantity that changes.' All changes occur in time (*Frege*, 1952; *Joseph*, 1973). Thus, in a univariant system, f is 1.0, and the fundamental process is the growth and development of the organism, as described by the synthesis of macromolecular colloidal substances.

Cells and tissues do not develop independently of one another. If the state of the organism is represented as a set of macromolecular subsets, then:

$$S = (M, N, O, P \ldots),$$

where S represents the physicochemical state of tissues denoted by the subsets, M, N, O, P, etc. Then if, for example, dielectric energy or dielectric constant in any tissue, P, are functions of neuromuscular synthesis (or of time):

$$(c_{Na}'' \, \Delta\mu_{Na}°) = f_1 \, (p_1, p_2, p_3 \ldots)$$

and

$$(D'')_p = f_2 \, (p_1, p_2, p_3 \ldots)$$

and so on, for any number of secondary properties.

Thus, S also implies the set of all necessary properties related to D'' and $c_{Na}'' \, \Delta\mu_{Na}°$. Thus:

$$S = (D_1'', D_2'', D_3'' \ldots)$$

Accordingly, the set of dielectric properties in each of the subsets (M, N, O, P ...) is highly coordinated by reciprocal biunivocal correspondences, and no member of the set of phases or tissue (P, for example) can develop independently of the others (M, N, O ...). It is this property derived from the phase rule, which unifies the organism, and causes it to develop with a sense or organicism (chapter 9). Thus, *Claude Bernard*'s science of general physiology acquires the 'organizing sense' from *Gibbs*' equilibrium of heterogeneous substances, or phase rule, by reason of which organisms relate behavior to morphology.

Development of the Organism as a Whole

As has been shown in tables I and II, the dielectric properties of skeletal muscle and brain in the human being can be described by reference to the dielectric constant D'' and to the acid-base balance between any two phases, as measured by the mean equivalent weight of the colloid, or by x, the density of colloidal charge, measured as Eq/kg water (*Joseph*, 1971a, b).

Electrolyte balance between intracellular and extracellular phases (or the *milieu intérieur*) is described by five ion concentrations of the form $(c_i'')/(c_i')$. Since the five extracellular concentrations are invariant in the standard state of any extracellular fluid, each intracellular concentration is given by an equation of the form:

$$\Delta\mu_i = \Delta\mu_i^\circ + RT \ln (r_i)'',$$

where the activity coefficient of each ion in the standard physiological state (homeostasis) is assigned the value of 1.0 (chapter 3). For each of the five kinds of ion, this yields an equation of the form:

$$\Delta\mu_i = (\Delta\mu_i^\circ)' + RT \ln (r_i),$$

where $\Delta\mu_i$ is the change of chemical potential, and $(\Delta\mu_i^\circ)'$ is the apparent change of standard chemical potential for any given kind of ion. This depends on the ionization constant α'' in the intracellular phase; this depends on the intracellular state of water, and is therefore to be regarded as a dielectric property, or a function of D''. Thus, each of the five values of $(\Delta\mu_i^\circ)'$ is a function of D'';

$$(\Delta\mu_i^\circ)' = f(D'') \text{ (five equations)}.$$

Also

$$\Delta\mu_{Na} = \Delta\mu_K = \frac{1}{2}\Delta\mu_{Ca} = \frac{1}{2}\Delta\mu_{Mg} = -\Delta\mu_{Cl} \text{ (four equations)}.$$

Thus, any given value of $\Delta\mu_i$ depends on the intracellular state of water, as given by D''. It also depends on the density of colloidal charge, x, through the relation for acid-base balance:

$$x + \Sigma (c_i)'' z_i = 0.$$

This yields a total of 15 equations among the following 15 parameters for five ions:

(1) $\Delta\mu_i$ (change of chemical potential; four equations).
(2) $(\Delta\mu_i^\circ)'$ five equations relating $(\Delta\mu_i^\circ)'$ to D''.
(3) (r_i) or $(c_i)''$ five equations relating $(\Delta\mu_i^\circ)'$ and $(c_i)''$.
(4) $\Sigma (c_i)''$ and x (one equation relating $(c_i)''$ to x, the colloidal charge).

There are therefore 15 independent equations relating 15 parameters: $\Delta\mu_i$, $(\Delta\mu_i^\circ)'$ and $(c_i)''$ for each of five ions. Let us assume that each of these depends only on the nature and total mass and ordering of n macromolecular components, which are functions of age and state of development of any given kind of cell or tissue. It is therefore a function of the time-dependent state of aggregation. Then it would follow that D'' and x, in the general case do not vary independently.

In this situation, a given kind of cell or tissue is characterized by only one degree of freedom, which represents its one possibility of growth or development as a function of time. At any given point on such a growth curve, such a cell or tissue shows a 'sense of organization' determined by its internal state of order, or 'negative entropy' of $(n + 6)$ substances. Here n represents the number of characteristic cellular macromolecules, and 6 represents water plus the five kinds of inorganic ions. In contrast to the n immobile macromolecular substances, water and the five physiological ions are subject to *reversible* transport. This is *Carnot*'s condition for an invariant heterogeneous system, in which isothermal cyclical work is zero. It is also the condition for stable heterogeneous distribution in a biological system containing $(n + 6)$ substances within any intracellular aggregate.

Aging Parameters

It has been shown in the preceding section that in any intracellular structure, water, and electrolyte balance is determined by the growth and development of an intracellular set of n macromolecular components that determine all the dielectric properties of the dispersion medium, intracellular water, as well as the necessary behavioral properties such as irritability, contractility, tension, work, and all other properties related to configurational entropy and free energy. The secondary properties should also be considered to include rates of respiratory metabolism and changes which also depend on the behavior of water as a polar or non-polar solvent (*Joseph,* 1973). Thus, cellular structures behave as well-ordered units in the sense understood by *Claude Bernard*, rather than as physicochemical mechanisms, explicable only by the principles of causality and sufficient reason, as current theories of 'active transport' would have it.

Well-ordered development of human morphology is therefore correlated with well-ordered development of behavior in the growth period of infants and children. It is in that period that children begin to acquire physiological and mental control of such essential qualities of adult behavior as speech, language, communication, and methods of locomotion, including artificial or mechanical. The development of the body may be studied by the chemistry of the *aging parameters,* as shown by table III. Essentially, two kinds of parameters are included: dielectric properties and acid-base balance. Since these are both functions of cell morphology, each type of property is age-dependent. There-

Table III. Aging parameters in pigs and men[1]

Tissue	Skeletal	Heart muscle	Liver	Brain	Kidney
Dielectric constant					
Man	Fetus	66	43	64	58	54
	Newborn	51	50	56	58	57
	Adult	31	50	49	58	65
Pig	Fetus	65	43	54	57	57
	Newborn	48	54	52	56	63
	Adult	28	44	43	57	58
Equivalent weight, g/equiv.					
Man	Fetus	1,140	1,600	2,070	1,370	1,480
	Newborn	2,520	2,170	3,430	1,880	1,670
	Adult	2,100	2,200	3,640	2,370	2,490
Pig	Fetus	1,040	1,210	2,160	1,210	1,010
	Newborn	2,000	1,660	2,250	1,450	1,580
	Adult	2,300	1,750	2,730	2,460	2,720
Dielectric energy, cal/kg H_2O					
Man	Fetus	36.58	73.78	32.24	49.49	61.96
	Newborn	71.30	74.40	53.32	61.24	60.05
	Adult	80.60	68.20	59.52	53.82	40.19
Pig	Fetus	41.40	70.68	55.56	60.05	54.55
	Newborn	71.92	83.88	56.42	61.72	42.10
	Adult	83.70	71.30	67.58	52.63	60.05

[1] From *Joseph* (1973).

fore, the two related sets of variables are never independent, and biological structures in the growth period are univariant, with one degree of freedom.

In table III, the following tissues are represented for human beings, as compared with pigs: skeletal muscle, heart, liver, brain, and kidney. In both man and pig, the greatest changes in the dielectric properties are found in the growth period of skeletal muscle. Thus, in the human being, the dielectric constant of skeletal muscle decreases from 66 to 31 between fetal and adult states. In the pig, the comparable values are 65 and 28. Thus, in both species there are marked changes in the state of intracellular water during the growth period.

The development of rat skeletal muscle from 2 to 65 days is shown in table II; between these two limits, the dielectric constant decreases from 68 to 28. In the same period, the change of standard chemical potential, $\Delta\mu_{Na}°$, increases from 0.37 to 3.32 kcal/mole; dielectric energy $c_{Na}{}'' \Delta\mu_{Na}{}°$ increases from 41.54 to 78.99 cal/kg water.

Thus, the set of three properties related to the dielectric properties of intracellular water increases during the growth period in many similar ways for three mammalian species: man, pig, and rat. The dielectric constant D'' is of the order of 65–68 in the fetal or early postpartum period; this approaches the value of liquid water, about 80. At the same time, the value of the dielectric energy is of the order of 40 cal/kg water, about half the adult values. Thus, skeletal muscle attains its full strength only after the end of the growth period, at which time the system becomes invariant rather than univariant, as in the growth period. Meanwhile the mean equivalent weight of the muscle colloid increases from values of the order of 1,000 g/equivalent to values that approximate 2,000 g, an increase of about 100%. This corresponds to an increase of about 100%. The ratio of nitrogen to phosphorus likewise increases by about 100%, accompanying the synthesis of contractile proteins, with little increase of the nucleic acids. The increase of equivalent weight is comparable to that observed in other types of tissue, where the adult values are generally observed to be of the order of 2,000–3,000 g/Eq. Thus, the rate of synthesis of the structural protoplasm is greater than that of the genetic type, as measured by either equivalent weight characteristic of nucleic acids. This is also indicated by a low ratio of nitrogen to phosphorus (*Joseph*, 1973).

Detailed comparison of the aging parameters for the five tissues shows the following points (table II):

(1) High dielectric constants in the fetal period occur not only in human skeletal muscle (66), but also in liver (64) and brain (58). In the pig, the corresponding fetal values are: skeletal muscle (65), brain (57), and kidney (57). In liver, the value is slightly lower (54). In fetal human heart, the value of D'' is 43; the same value is found in fetal pig heart.

(2) In the development of skeletal muscle from the fetal to the adult state, there are large decreases both in human beings and in the pig. In the adult human, the value of D'' is 31; in the adult pig, D'' is 28. This is also about the value calculated for the 65-day rat (table II).

(3) In the other four tissues (heart, liver, brain, and kidney, there are no changes of D'' that are comparable to those found in skeletal muscle. Thus, in the human heart, the change of D'' is about 43–50. In liver, the range is from 61 to 49. In brain the value of D'' remains constant at 58, and in kidney, the range of variation is from 51 to 65.

In the pig, the range of variation in heart, liver, kidney, and brain is generally in the same range as the values found for D'' in human beings and the aging changes are small, as compared with those for skeletal muscle.

(4) Dielectric energy in both man and pig shows systematic increases of the order of 100% in skeletal muscle as it develops. In both species, the value in fetal

skeletal muscle is of the order of 40 cal/kg water, as compared with values of about 80 cal in the adult. The increase of $c_{Na}'' \Delta\mu_{Na}°$ in the rat is of the same order of magnitude from the age of 2 days until 65 days (table II).

(5) No comparable aging changes of dielectric energy are found in the other four tissues. In human tissues, the levels of dielectric energy remain within the following ranges:

Heart	68.20–74.40 cal/kg water
Liver	32.24–58.52 cal/kg water
Brain	49.49–62.24 cal/kg water
Kidney	40.19–61.96 cal/kg water

At all ages, with one exception, the dielectric energy remains high (40 cal or higher), but with the exception of skeletal muscle, heart shows the highest values of dielectric energy (about 70 cal at all ages), as compared with 80 cal for adult skeletal muscle. This can be related to the contractile functions of both muscular tissues, which in the adult state maintain high configurational free energy, low configurational entropy, and low dielectric constants, characteristic of well-organized states of water. These properties are highly dependent on growth and aging of skeletal muscle, but much less so in heart, which must be highly functional at all ages from fetal to adult states.

As is also the case with the dielectric properties of the intracellular state of water, acid-base balance in any kind of cell or tissue is dependent on age as well as on the nature of the tissue. This is shown in the following tabulations which compare the mean equivalent weights of five different tissues for human beings at the upper and lower limits (table III).

	Mean equivalent weight, g/Eq
Skeletal muscle	1,140–2,520
Heart	1,600–2,200
Liver	2,070–3,640
Brain	1,370–2,370
Kidney	1,480–2,490
Average	1,530–2,640

At the lower limit, values for each tissue occur in the fetus. At this level, the low equivalent weight is explained by the high ratio of nucleoproteins and nucleic acids to total colloid. This represents an increase in the amount of structural proteins during growth, referred to the genetic or chromosomal material, which predominates in the fetus. Synthesis related to an increase of the ratio of nitrogen to phosphorus corresponds to an increase of the mean equivalent weight of the cellular colloids.

Comparing the five different types of tissue, the highest values of the mean equivalent weight are found in liver, both in the fetus and in the adult. This would point to a difference in the intracellular proteins, characterized by a higher isoelectric point and a lowered base-binding capacity or net negative charge per unit weight.

The mean value of the colloidal equivalent weight is 1,530 g/Eq in the fetus and 2,640 g/Eq in the postpartum or adult period. As in the case of liver, this increase in the growth period can be related to the increased synthesis of nitrogen-rich structural proteins of higher isoelectric points than those of nucleic acids or nucleoproteins. The greatest increase of equivalent weight therefore occurs in skeletal muscle, which increases strongly in the growth period; this is required to meet the functional needs of muscular tissue with respect to work and tension. Thus, the mean equivalent weight of the muscle colloids increases from 1,140 to 2,580 g/Eq — a factor of 120%. For heart, the increase is from 1,600 to 2,200 g/Eq, an increase of less than 40%. The dielectric properties of heart muscle, D'', $\Delta\mu_{Na}°$, and c_{Na}'' $\Delta\mu_{Na}°$, also tend to remain fairly independent of age, as compared with skeletal muscle. This is true also for the properties of liver, brain, and kidney (table III). Thus, among the five developing tissues, only skeletal muscle shows striking age changes of dielectric properties. These include dielectric energy, which is required to meet the age-dependent functions of tension and work. Development of these properties is also conspicuous in the other tissues, which are functional in all fetal and post-partum periods, as well as in the later stages of life. Thus, at all stages of the life span, behavior depends on the morphological properties of cells and tissues with respect to dielectric properties of cells and tissues with respect to hydration energies and acid-base balance, as reflected by the synthesis of structural proteins.

According to the results of table III, skeletal muscle, heart, liver, kidney, and brain develop independently, but according to general principles of growth and aging. Thus, if S is the set of all organs, tissues and protoplasmic structures in the organism:

$$S = (M, N, O, P ...)$$

where M denotes the set of all myofibrils, N the set of all neurones, O the set of all visceral organs, and P the set of all cardiovascular structures (heart, arteries, veins, and capillaries). Then S is the set of all structures that constitute the histochemical or protoplasmic morphology of the body. Then the general law of the body requires that there be biunivocal correspondences between any of the subsets M, N, O, P ... as they develop in time over any given period.

Then the electrolyte-water composition of any type of cell or tissue depends on growth and development, as determined by chemical morphology (*Joseph,* 1973). Thus, if the potassium concentration $(c_K)''$, for example, in any myofibril is a function of morphology,

$$(c_K)'' = f_1 \ (p_1, p_2 \ ...),$$

where p_1, p_2 ... denote the composition of the interfibrillar set of proteins, then:

$$S = f_2 \ ([c_K]'' \ ...).$$

Similar relations hold for all protoplasmic structural units. Then all cells and tissues, with respect to intracellular electrolytes, are characterized by biunivocal correspondences between any pair of subsets (M, N, O, P ...). Accordingly, all growth rates of individual cells and tissues are coordinated by one-to-one correspondences between all subsets of protoplasmic structures. This corresponds at any time to morphological 'firstness' of the organism. It is described for certain human and mammalian tissues in tables I—III. At any particular point on the growth curve, behavior depends on energies and potentials of entire groups or sets of morphological structures. Therefore, 'secondness' as a function of age, growth, and development is synechistic or 'held together' with firstness.

Especially in human beings, secondness and firstness, as they develop synechistically in time, imply the properties of 'thirdness', which imply extension in time (chapter 1). These properties imply everything related to the development of reason, mind, and purposeful behavior. These properties, as was early discerned by *Locke* in 1690, depend on *a postiori* experience, and are therefore both well-ordered and pluralistic (chapters 4 and 8). They develop rapidly, especially in the growth period of children, and are directly related to and synechistic with the well-ordered set S that describes firstness (tables I—III).

Psychological Development of Children

According to the results of chapter 4 ('understanding'), the following human faculties represent a small group of components of 'human understanding' (*Locke,* 1968). (1) Ideas of logic. (2) Reason. (3) Ideas of number. (4) Association of ideas. (5) Space, time, and motion. (6) Ideas of chance, probability, and law.

Many other aspects of human reason, behavior and understanding may be included, extending the list indefinitely.

All these faculties are aspects of thirdness, and begin to develop in very early periods of childhood or infancy. Modern experience confirms *Locke* in the opinion that all knowledge is basically empirical and *a postiori*. None is congenital or acquired by genetic inheritance.

The above list of six aspects of thirdness suggests problems for experimental observations on young children of various ages, carried out under controlled conditions. Such observations have been carried out by *Piaget* and his collaborators, among others within about the last 50 years. It would carry one far afield to attempt to describe the results in detail. Hence, it must suffice merely to enumerate a short list of titles, which suggest the present status of *Piaget*'s studies in this field as a basis for further elaboration of the problem of mental growth and development.

It should be noted that the theories of education implied in these studies are of the nature of Jamesian introspection and of *Koehler*'s gestalt psychology rather than of behaviorist or reflex physiological psychology. The problem can thus be regarded as one of organicism (chapter 9) or of structuralism (chapters 1 and 12) rather than of Cartesian dualistic mechanism (chapter 2).

The following works of *Piaget* may be cited:

1   *Piaget, J. and Inholder, B.:* The psychology of the child (Basic Books, New York 1969).
2   *Piaget, J.:* The principles of genetic epistemology (Basic Books, New York 1972).
3   *Piaget, J.:* Science of education and the psychology of the child (Orion Press, New York 1970).
4   *Piaget, J.:* Main trends in psychology (Harper & Row, London 1973).
5   *Piaget, J. and Inholder, B.:* The origin of the idea of chance in children (Norton, New York 1975).

Chapter 11

Philosophical Anthropology

Two well-known quotations (*Pope* and *Protagoras*) provide an adequate basis for the subject of philosophical anthropology: 'the proper study of mankind is man' — *Alexander Pope* in *Essay on Man* (18th century); 'man is the measure of all things' — *Protagoras* (5th century, BC). These quotations affirm an underlying continuous reiteration of anthropocentric or anthropomorphic bases for all human efforts in philosophy, literature, history, and archaeology ever since these subjects attained organized expression.

The modern science of anthropology attained the basis for its present mature status in the 19th century period of *Darwin* and *Huxley*. The modern point of view is fully illustrated by the title of *Huxley*'s book *Man's Place in Nature* (1863). Here human beings are frankly treated as members of the order of Primates, along with related species such as the higher apes (the gorilla, the orangoutang and the chimpanzee). Thus, the human species is studied as a member of a phylogenetically related group that includes such diversified species as the lemur, the gibbon and the higher apes. These species were recognized by *Linnaeus* (1751) to comprise a closely related group with similar anatomical, morphological, and physiological characteristics common to man and the chimpanzee. Many such physicochemical characteristics are common to larger and widely varying groups of mammals and cold-blooded vertebrates, as well as to invertebrates (*Joseph, 1973*).

Since the publication of *Man's Place in Nature* in 1863, the ensuing researches in fossilized and surviving species of the primates of the Old World continents (Europe, Asia, and South Africa), have led to a greatly increased knowledge of the evolution and geographical distribution of all known species and varieties. For example, modern students of primatology are now cognizant of the increased range of structure and behavior in monkeys. Living families show various types arrested at definite fossilized stages, followed by later phylogenetic stages, becoming stabilized at various succeeding levels represented by living species of Old and New World monkeys. These stages are represented, for example, by the development of stereoscopic vision, by the evolution of prehensile hands and feet, the expansion of the brain, the extension of longevity, changes of dentition, and related structures of the oral cavity; all such changes have been coordinated at rates that are characteristic of each special group or subgroup of monkeys in various parts of the world. These processes, since the time of *Huxley*, have become evident in the geological record revealed by fossilized remains and other paleontological evidence. The end-results of the evolutionary process are now manifested by the anatomical structure and physiological behavior of living species, including the higher apes and man.

The fact that the several types of changes have been occurring independently in various groups of Old and New World monkeys has been regarded as remarkable by paleontologists and primatologists. Since the separation of the groups occurred soon after their origin in the Eocene period, the various lines of development have been remarkably parallel.

For example, groups of Old World apes and New World spider monkeys have developed independently the mode of locomotion known as brachiation, whereby the animal swings from branch to branch by extremely long movements of the arms. Obviously, these parallel and independent changes of behavior habits among different species that occupy widely separated geographical habitats are analogous to similar changes observed among widely distributed human groups, ranging from Africa or the Middle East to Mexico or Peru in the human historical record. Thus, both anthropological and anthropoidal behavior are known to develop along parallel lines among species or races that are genetically related only by extremely distant time relationships.

Man's Predecessors

The ancestors of the human race seem to have separated from ape-like predecessors about 20 million years ago in the Miocene. This occurred somewhere in one of the three Old World continents. However, the earliest fossil forms of these human forerunners seem to have been confined to East Africa, and to date from periods of 0.5 to 2 million years ago. They were first discovered in 1923 in the neighborhood of Johannesburg by *Raymond Dart;* discoveries in other parts of Africa occurred somewhat later. Several significant advances in primitive behavior have been attributed to these prehuman types: (1) the use of tools fashioned from bone, horn and stone; (2) development of the teeth toward the human state; (3) approach to an upright posture, and (4) retention of the small 'ape-like' brain capacity.

Several competing species seem to have been identifiable, not belonging to a well-evolved uniform type. These earliest forms of man seem to have abandoned the forests and to have attained characteristic omnivorous habits. Different competing forms seem to have evolved parallel lines of development in varying habitats. Omnivorous forms seem to have survived at the expense of more highly vegetarian varieties. In general, development occurred toward the evolution of agricultural rather than arboreal forms of life. Thus, climbing forms of locomotion were gradually abandoned in favor of erect, vertical bipedal locomotion. In accordance with a slow tempo of anatomical evolution, early human forms were also characterized by slow rates of behavioral change. The early forms of tools and locomotion were retained for long periods in all habitats.

A number of questions have arisen as a result of continued research on the nature of human evolution since *Huxley*'s *Man's Place in Nature*. It has been agreed that there have recurred during a period of 0.5 million years a great enlargement and improvement in the human brain in all the geographical races of man. Evolutionary development has been both parallel and divergent, occurring at different tempi and rates, depending on phylogenetic and chronological factors. The first geographical races, arising in East Africa, in Java, in China, and in certain regions of western Europe, may possibly be regarded as the forerunners of the modern races, depending on comparative chronology. This was the suggestion offered by *Waldenreich* (1924), and supported by *Coon*. Evidence points to continual divergence in the development of human structures in Chinese and European peoples.

A rather difficult and detailed study of *Tempi and Mode in Evolution* (*Simpson*, 1965) illustrates some of the more significant factors that may be involved in results such as the foregoing, relating to parallel and divergent evolution in various species. Among these factors are rates of mutation, size and density of population, and the statistical variability within any given population at any given time. Lamarckism (inheritance of acquired characteristics) and vitalism (or teleological purposefulness) may be definitely excluded, leaving only natural selection, rates of mutation, and stability of the gene as the decisive factors (*Schrodinger*, after *Delbruck*, 1944; *Joseph*, 1973). Mutation rates are related to rates of isomerization, depending on activation energies of internal molecular rearrangements.

'Selection is a vector having intensity and direction' (*Simpson*, 1965). Direction of selection can be analyzed into three components: centrifugal, centripetal, and linear. The first tends to cause spreading or divergence, the second tends to concentrate a population about a nodal point, and the third tends to cause a shift of the nodal point. These are, of course, rather crude but useful generalizations. However, they tend to describe the main factual outlines of human development in the four main types deriving from East Africa, Java, Pekin, and Western Europe. The main human stocks have developed at different tempi and modes, and with varying degrees of divergence and linearity. The role of teleology or transcendent purposefulness may probably continue in a realm of non-scientific speculation beyond the accessibility of any conceivable experimental or observational approach.

In the preceding pages, we have dealt mainly with the subject of physical anthropology, which is concerned with the development of social, cultural, and geological forms of human behavior. When all aspects of human life, thought, and behavior are considered in their totality at all periods, in all species and geographical locations, we may approach a general view of *Man's Place in Nature,* finally attaining a comprehensive grasp of what is comprised by the term 'philosophical anthropology'.

The general subject may be approached from the most elementary or primitive requirements of the early races of man. These included the use of tools and weapons, as they were required in agriculture, hunting and defense. The most elementary requirements of all societies are nutritional, reproductive, shelter, and defense. Tools and weapons were required at all social and cultural levels to satisfy these elementary needs. In the course of time, various of the decorative arts were evolved to embellish these elementary needs such as tools, weapons, and habitations. These required increased manual skills and dexterity, and were refined appeals to the sense organs. They also required developments of speech, vocal communication, and the use of language, all of which were related to changed conditions of physical anthropology. Thus, over the entire range of human evolution, physical and cultural anthropology are inseparable. It is only over relatively short periods of history that cultural and social development can be studied independently of physical changes; this requires a full and complete stabilization of the genetic characterization of any human group.

Whatever may have been the genetic mechanisms of human evolution, it is quite certain that the development of the skull and brain that led to the perfection of the human speech apparatus was of central importance to survival (*du Brul,* 1958). The evolutionary processes and morphological changes were essential to the well-ordered adaptations that led to the numerous languages and dialects now spoken in various parts of the earth.

Evidently, thousands of generations of human evolution dating from the earliest fossil remains were required to stabilize human anatomy, and especially the size and shape of the skull characteristic of contemporary races. Adaptation of the skull to the evolution of upright posture and the development of the hands and arms have been studied by *Waldenreich* (1924) and by *du Brul and Sicher* (1954). The concomitant development of the oral cavity and teeth along with the vocal cords were essential to the development of human speech. This added a second auxiliary function to those of the initial feeding, mastication, and digestive processes. These developments of brain, skull, arms, forearms, and hands preceded the development of digital and manual skills, and would also have preceded the evolution of sensations, perceptions, and esthetic feelings and faculties. These are essential to the full development of all the varied manifestations of cultural anthropology.

In all the manifestations of anthropological evolution in the physical sense, two main types of vital processes may be distinguished (*Joseph,* 1973). These include reversible processes that are required to maintain invariant internal conditions within each organism over the entire phylogenetic and ontogenetic succession of changes. An example is the preservation of a constant *milieu intérieur* in all species of mammals at all periods of the life span (*Bernard,* 1878). It has been shown that the characteristic concentrations of the various cations of the *milieu intérieur* maintain certain constant features common to all living mammals: these characteristics point to a common origin in primitive sea water (*Macallum,* 1910, 1926; *Joseph,* 1973).

Thus, the chemical potential of water in all cells and tissues of mammals remains constant at all stages of the life span. The value corresponds to a constant freezing point depression, Δ, of blood plasma of the order of $-0.58\,°C$. This corresponds to a value of -3.05 cal/mole as referred to the value of $0\,°C$. Thus:

$$\mu_{H_2O} - \mu_{H_2O}° = 5.26\,\Delta\ \text{cal/mole,}$$

where 5.26 cal/mole/degree is the entropy of fusion of ice.

Thus, as a first approximation, the chemical potentials of water and of the physiological electrolytes, NaCl, KCl, $CaCl_2$, and $MgCl_2$ remain constant in all mammalian cells and tissues, independently of species, age, growth, and development. They are ontogenetic and phylogenetic invariants. As thermodynamic functions, the five chemical potentials listed above are classed as *zero order* functions. They are independent of total mass, size, shape, or function of any kind of structure. They are therefore non-adaptive functions.

In contrast to the non-adaptive zero order functions listed above, there are the first order adaptive functions related to total mass, volume, size, and shape of any structure or set of structures. These functions would then include all changes of posture, development of skull, forearm and appendages, and all the physical functions that depend only on growth, form, entropy and phylogeny. Behavior therefore should be classified among the first order functions. It can evolve over geological epochs under conditions in which the 'firstness' of protoplasm remains unchanged.

Linguistics

Language at any time or place is one of the best reflections we have of human behavior at all levels — practical, social, religious, scientific, or philosophical. At any stage of history, language is inseparably bound to the life of any people. It has previously been explained that the development of language depends on the morphological evolution of the skull, the mouth, lips, tongue, and cheeks, and other structures of the oral cavity, as well as on the formation of vocal cords, which vibrate in resonance with the throat and upper respiratory passages.

The energy of human speech is generated by passage of air from the lungs.

The main systems of branching tubes conducting expired air from the lungs meet in the wind pipe or trachea. In the adult human being, this is an air tube about 2 cm in diameter and 20 cm in length. At the upper end, the trachea leads to the larynx. The system is flexible, and is supported by a strongly cartilagenous structure at the circumference. At the larynx, the shape of the windpipe changes from cylindrical to a flattened form. The vocal cords connected with the windpipe are contained within a muscular structure shaped like the lips of the mouth, but considerably smaller. The muscular structures of the vocal cords lie across the upper flattened part of the trachea, and contain the vibrating cords.

The pitch of the voice is determined by the tension of the muscular tissue, which determines the frequency of the vibrations of the voice. The pitch ranges from one corresponding to a frequency of about 60/sec (low bass) to one of about 1,300/sec (high soprano).

As has been shown in chapter 3, the tension of a muscle is proportional to its dielectric energy, expressed in joules or in cal/kg water. Thus:

$$- t = + 8.60 \, c_{Na}{}'' \, \Delta\mu_{Na}{}°,$$
$$= 3,000 \, g/cm^2.$$

When $c_{Na}{}'' \, \Delta\mu_{Na}{}°$ is 80 cal or 335 j/kg water, E_a in millivolts is given by the formula:

$$t = 830 \, c_{Na}{}'' \, E_a.$$

The pitch of the voice, as measured by the frequency of the vibrations, is proportional to the tension of the vocal cords, which has been roughly measured for various ranges of the human voice from bass to soprano (*von Helmholtz,* 1862, 1954). The frequency and pitch of the musical tones are controlled by the tension of the vocal cords, which depends on the dielectric energy of the muscle fibers, which are thus under voluntary control. Increasing the pitch of the voice by one octave implies an increase of the dielectric energy and tension by a factor of two. This conforms to a law discovered by *Pythagoras* and other ancient Greek mathematicians, and studied experimentally by an instrument, the *monochord,* which proved that pitch was inversely proportional to the length of a vibrating string. This law is fundamental in musical theory, and was confirmed by *d'Alembert, Galileo,* and other theorists of modern times. It is essential as the theoretical basis for the tuning of stringed instruments, including the harpsichord and pianoforte. Vocal communication among human beings thus depends on a fundamental law of physiological acoustics. Many other physical principles enter into the pronunciation of words and the enunciation of sentences. These principles are among those governing the use of speech and language in all human groups, subgroups or tribes, and are thus fundamental in the study of cultural anthropology.

The foregoing principles applied to the evolutionary factors related to the development of speech and language can be isolated from the various aspects of cultural anthropology, and related primarily to physical anthropology as it describes the evolution of the skull, mouth parts, and oral cavity in general without regard to specific cultural factors. Given the full acquisition of stable phylogenetic characters, as determined by the zero order and first order thermodynamic and genetic functions, the origins and development of language follow separate parallel or divergent evolutionary lines on a geologal or geophysical time scale according to the three main modes and tempi of evolution, as previously outlined: parallel, linear, or divergent. These various modes are related to all other changes of cultural and ethological behavior in the various races of man. As previously noted, language is possibly the best indication of the total life and culture of any human group at any given period in its history. When fully developed and mature, it reflects the history, politics, sociology, literature, religion, and philosophy of any period. In western cultures, it has attained full maturity among the ancient Greeks, the Hebrews, and the Romans, for example.

In these early cultures, the study of rhetoric was already well developed, and required in the education of the youth of the privileged classes. Thus, in very early times, the rules of grammatical expression had been fully formulated, and the principles of linguistics proper to the time and place had been established. At any period, these principles were fundamental in philosophical anthropology, regardless of the nature of the people or social group to which they were applied. Thus, the rules of grammar and rhetoric were required in the education of the learned with regard to the ancient languages, Greek, Latin, Hebrew, and Arabic, as well as to the developing languages of modern Europe — English, French, Italian, and Spanish. Among specialists, this led to the study of comparative linguistics and ethnology. It can be extended to include any language, modern, medieval, or ancient, in any part of the world. Studies of this nature are necessary parts of the linguistic training of professional anthropologists, depending on the nature of the human groups which form the field of their major interests.

Thus, the field of linguistics can be and has been approached from many points of view — anthropological, comparative, historical, psychological, and philosophical. It should be realized that language, speech, and communication are all based on the morphological and physiological development of the human being, beginning in childhood and continuing over the entire life span. Language in the child is learned from the parents and the schools; it is therefore a continuous cultural heritage that unifies and coordinates all human societies, homogeneous and heterogeneous. This was well understood by philosophers of the enlightenment, such as *Locke,* who in his *Essay on Human Understanding* buttressed his anthropological and anthropocentric principles with arguments based on the use of language. At all other periods, thinkers have regarded language as inseparable from thought and reason; it is therefore at the foundation of all human knowledge, thought, and reason.

Origin and Structure of Language

Modern research in cultural anthropology seems to have shown that many primitive cultures (and many relatively advanced cultures) have adhered to a belief in the divine origin of language. According to the *Book of Genesis,* for example, 'And the Lord God having formed out of the ground all the beasts of the earth and all the fowls of the air, brought them to Adam to see what he would call them; for whatsoever Adam called any living creature, the same is its name.' Similar beliefs in the divine origin of language were held by the Egyptians, Babylonians, Chinese, Hindus, and Icelandic peoples. This is easily understood from a more generally widespread belief that all human institutions, beliefs, and customs, whether religious or secular, were of divine origin. Primitive beliefs of this kind must have necessarily been prevalent in historical periods where *causality* or *sufficient reason* rather than *natural law* were the normal modes of explanation (chapter 6). It is only in modern post-renaissance or post-scholastic modes of rational or empiricist thought that anthropological modes of explanation in relation to all aspects of cultural and philosophical anthropology occur.

Comparative Philology

Linguistic studies during the 19th century were directed for the most part by the methods of comparative philology. This approach is mainly concerned with the study of the history of languages, as related to the origin of words and their meaning ('etymology'). However, this definition is inadequate and misleading, for the origins and development of words comprise but a small part of the subject matter of comparative philology. As the study of languages developed over the past few centuries in actual practice, there arose a rather wide gap between those scholars who considered themselves as philologists and a group known rather as linguists. The latter group included those mainly interested in the structure of language from the point of view of grammar. Those known as philologists were interested mainly in historical questions and in problems of etymology rather than of grammar. The problems relating to this dualistic aspect of language studies might seem to be related to questions of emphasis rather than to any actual antagonism of the two points of view. In the 20th century, competent linguists appear to be equally interested in questions of structure and grammar as well as in those of history and philology.

The study of comparative philology as a science required the close scrutiny of various languages with regard to their similarities in grammar and syntax. In earlier times, little attention seems to have been directed toward the uniformities that underly each language of a common group with respect to structure, syntax, and grammar. These similarities and regularities often tended to be overlooked by those linguists who were interested mainly in historic or philological development.

In addition to questions of grammar and syntax as related to historical development, the science of philology is also concerned with the mechanisms of oral speech, as described by *phonetics, phonology,* and *morphology.* The subject of phonetics for centuries has been a matter of interest to everyone professionally engaged in the subject of public speaking. This would include actors, orators, elocutionists, and language teachers interested in the principles of correct pronunciation and diction. Correct or eloquent speech is based on the physiology of the mouth parts, throat, vocal cords, and oral cavity. Pronunciation and accenting depend on understanding of the nature of vowels, consonants, whisperings, and a great variety of other vocal sounds, and on the principles of pitch, resonance, and rhythm. Thus, considered as an art of elocution, speech and diction as taught by professionals in the science of phonetics have, at any level of quality, a physiological basis. Well-controlled or eloquent speech implies perfect control of breathing, respiration, and voluntary control of the mouth, vocal cords, and oral cavity.

The subject of phonetics is also occupied with methods of conveying the actual sound of spoken language, as distinguished from *written* language. Sounds can often be conveyed in written language by authors with sufficient skill to transcribe the actual vocal sounds by ingenious forms of spelling. *Mark Twain,* for example was able by clever spelling and punctuation to convey the actual vocal sounds produced by a great number of characters in *Huckleberry Finn* who represented a wide variety of dialects and accents found along the Mississippi in the states of Missouri, Kentucky, Arkansas, and Mississippi. He cultivated the mastery of vocal and written phonetics in his many years as a pilot on Mississippi steamboats, acquiring an extremely sensitive skill in transmitting the actual vocal characteristics of a great variety of peoples of all the region, including slaves, men, women, and children of all types, thus creating a permanently valid picture of American life before the Civil War. This is an example of the practical value of phonetics as a record of actual life. (Incidentally, the very large number of Americanisms in *Huckleberry Finn* have been successfully translated into the French language. Obviously, skillful use of phonetic principles can be applied to the promotion of international understanding and good will among all educated people of all lands.)

There are great differences in the spoken use of the English language as actually pronounced and understood by inhabitants of various regions of the United States. This of course is a matter of great interest not only to professional writers and dramatists, but also to philologists. Eminent writers for the stage, such as *Bernard Shaw* in *Pygmalion,* who included a professional philologist *(Henry Higgins)* as a protagonist, have depicted with great humor and human interest, the linguistic problems involved in the social class distinctions in London society. The main linguistic problem is the phonetic and grammatical one of elevating the speech and behavior of a slum girl from London (one *Liza Doolittle*) to the level of elegance required of a lady of the upper classes. *Shaw,* as an Irishman, was acutely sensitive to every nuance of English class society as reflected in phonetics, grammar, and behavior. These distinctions are not so much physical or genetic as they are social, cultural, and anthropological. They cannot be separated from the structure of free expression of thought and feeling, as well as for the functioning of the creative imagination. Similarly, much substantive discussion of grammar throughout the development of what we have been calling 'Cartesian linguistics' derives from this assumption (*Chomsky,* 1966).

Certain linguists reason from a postulated direct connection between language and mental processes in all participants in verbal discourse. This would seem to presuppose an introspective type of psychology in which a given speaker assumes that his own thoughts are accessible not only to himself, but to all the auditors, once they learned a common language or *universe of discourse.* Thus, the subjects of language and logic are unified by Cartesian linguistics or deep syntax by the nature of the human mind. Accordingly, it is necessary to adopt a view of language identical to that of the medieval realists, who presupposed the concrete reality and existence of linguistic universals. As *Levi-Strauss* (1970) has shown, this view of language is also held by many tribes of North American Indians.

As opposed to the medieval realists, nominalists of the type of *Abelard* and *Occam* tended to deny the objective reality of universals and to insist that each individual fact or object existed only in itself. For long periods of history, this seemed to have been the necessary basis for experimental science with its emphasis on objective, taxonomic and inductive methods. As an extreme tendency, this has led in modern times to various forms of positivism, which tend to deny the reality of intuitive human subjective *values.* Thus, Cartesian linguistics tend to affirm the validity of human value judgements obtained by introspection. Surface syntax or taxonomic linguistics, on the other hand, tend to favor a behaviorist or experimental type of psychology, in which only observable or experimental observations are permitted. Intuitive inferences tend to be excluded. Thus, one could imagine two observers witnessing the same experiment expressing the results as follows: (1) the rat *ate* the food pellet (behaviorist psychology, surface or taxonomic syntax, positivist metaphysics); (2) the rat *enjoyed* the pellet (introspective psychology, deep or Cartesian syntax, classical or 'humanist' metaphysics).

The type of metaphysics that is dominant in any human society at any time or place depends to a large extent on the fundamental social and economic values which are prevalent. In terms of Freudian psychology, this depends on the relative strength of the reality principle as compared with the pleasure principle. The reality principle requires only surface syntax to serve the linguistic needs of most people; the requirements of society at all levels require deep syntax of the creative elements of society. These depend on emotionally felt value judgements as well as on practical or technical judgements.

Zero-Order Functions

According to previously developed principles (chapters 3 and 4), the chemical potentials of water and the four electrolytes ($NaCl$, KCl, $CaCl_2$, $MgCl_2$) are zero-order functions. Therefore, in the primates, as in all other mammals, they are invariant and non-adaptive functions that establish the water and electrolyte composition of all the well-ordered phases of somatic cells as well as the composition and chemical potentials of water and electrolyte components of the *milieu intérieur*. In contrast to these five invariant zero-order functions, all thermodynamic functions related to the size, shape, anatomical organization, and biological functions of the evolving mammal or primate are first order and adaptive. These would include the size and shape of the skull and mouth parts, the dimensions and shape of arms, legs, hands, and feet, the methods of locomotion, and in man the evolution of speech, language and *cultural* rather than physical anthropology.

After the stabilization of the anatomical and physiological characteristics of any of the races of man, the only functions that are free to develop or evolve, or to retrogress, are the factors of cultural evolution, relating to behavior and values. These factors would therefore include the deep rather than the surface aspects of language. From the point of view of human psychology, only the introspectivist or 'value judgement' aspects are free to evolve; the behaviorist, mechanist, and reflex aspects of language would be fixed for all time by the constraints of a non-evolving zero-order set of physiological functions. Human evolution would then be restricted to a 'will to power' in Nietzschean forms of advancement, rather than to predetermined, mechanistic forms restricted by stabilized anatomical structure and reflex or behaviorist psychology.

According to the introspectivist psychology of *William James* or the objective idealism of *Peirce* (chapter 8), future human developments would be unrestricted by positivist limitations on human values. Radical empiricism and objective idealism represent a reformulation of the 18th century empiricism of *Locke* and *Hume*. They represent an attack on the strict materialism of positivism that assumes the possibility of eliminating a physiology of sensation, perception, and the phenomenology of will, emotions, and value judgements. Thus, the aims of *James'* radical empiricism and philosophical pluralism, like those of *Peirce*'s objective idealism, are consonant with the principles of physiological organicism (chapter 9) and with those of *Schopenhauer*'s voluntarism (chapter 7). They are incompatible with the principles of so-called mechanistic physiology, which would limit psychology and behavior to rather simple forms of tropisms, forced movements and reflexes, characteristic of simple forms of organization at lower levels of evolution.

Structural and Functional Anthropology

Structural anthropology, as a scientific discipline, is a rather recent development in the field of comparative cultural anthropology. It has been mainly associated with the work of *Levi-Strauss,* as expressed in his work *Structural Anthropology* (1963), and in certain other titles including *The Savage Mind* (1966). Structural anthropology, as the name implies, concerns itself mainly with the comparative study of social organization, or of various social orders, with reference to such subjects as kinship, mythology, language, religious beliefs, and ritual. As a comparative matter, primitive societies can be differentiated and classified according to various principles.

Applied Anthropology

The discipline presently known as applied anthropology came into existence in about the third and fourth decades of the 20th century (about 1920–1940) as a result of certain kinds of problems arising in the political and social life of that period. An earlier field of study was known as 'practical anthropology'. No sharp lines of distinction need be drawn between the various fields of cultural, social, and practical anthropology. All are related by the general subject of structural anthropology, dealing with problems of kinship, language, aging, and religious rites within any society or section of society. They are also related to problems of functional anthropology, as they deal with production of agricultural products, tools, weaponry, or other material necessities of life. The general problems of cultural anthropology were dealt with many years ago by *Sumner* in *Folkways* (1906), who studied the nature of mores in any section of society. The subject has also been treated in the treatise *Science of Society* by *Sumner* and *Keller.*

The emphasis of applied anthropology is placed on the study of social changes as they relate to changes of methods of production or distribution of material goods or commodities in any capitalist or socialist society.

These necessarily require coordinated changes by adaptations, not only in the society as a whole, but also deep and surface adaptations to a socialist structure in Soviet Russia, and the evolutionary change to a 'post-industrial' technological society. This has brought about increases in the populations of engineers, scientists, technologists and managers, and a relative diminution in the numbers the unskilled and illiterate classes. These changes in population have led to many changes in language, literature, and in the arts and sciences. Resistance to social and technological changes is always encountered in certain sections of the population that have been 'encultured' or deeply habituated to certain long-established folkways and traditions. Cultural and functional changes require processes of 'acculturation', or adaptations to new conditions of life. The rates of social and technological change have accelerated everywhere in the world in the 20th century. This has given rise to obvious in acculturation and reeducation at large of the human population on a universal scale. The problems require a widespread development of the sciences of applied and functional anthropology in future times. In many fields of study, traditional methods of education may no longer be adequate.

Primate Morphology

At the present period of human history, human anatomy and morphology have probably reached a point at which not only the zero-order functions of chemical morphology, chemical composition, and chemical potentials have been completely stabilized on both an ontological and phylogenetic basis, but also the first-order functions of size, shape and physiological development. These include brain weight, size, and anatomy of the skull, as well as neuromuscular development of all parts of the body.

The same may be said of numerous other species of primates, including the higher apes. In many respects, these are almost indistinguishable from man in physicochemical and physiological characteristics. The great difference is found in spiritual and mental characteristics, which result in a tremendous gap between man and all other primates. This gap has widened over the course of millions of years of evolution, during which the apes have remained at stationary levels in all respects, whereas man has retained only the primitive non-adaptive *milieu intérieur,* while advancing or retrogressing in all the first-order thermodynamic functions related to *physical* anthropology.

Nevertheless, the cultural adaptations of man appear to be almost limitless. These will be required to solve the innumerable problems that may be expected to arise in the next million years (*Peirce,* 1955). This is a measure of the stability of human genes and chromosomes, as well as the almost immeasurable stability of the species. Studies of comparative primatology on the basis of neuromuscular structure and 'molecular biology' have facilitated in certain species the development of quantitative evolutionary or phylogenetic divergence of any two related species. In the primates, for instance, this comparison can be made on the basis of the DNA base sequences of various species, including the chimpanzee and man (*King and Wilson,* 1975).

Other methods of studying genetic differences involve physicochemical, immunological, and sequencing studies of bases in the nucleic acids. All these methods have been applied to the study of the genetic distance between the chimpanzee *(Pan troglodytes)* and man *(Homo sapiens).* The two species have also been thoroughly compared at both genetic (molecular biological) and organizational levels.

King and Wilson have reported comparisons of amino acid sequence in twelve different polypeptides of man and chimpanzee. Only three of these showed significant differences between the two species. These were carbonic anhydrase, serum albumin, and transferrin. Such important proteins as the myoglobulin of muscle and the hemoglobins were practically identical. Thus, the proteins of man and chimpanzee, with few exceptions, remain largely identical on the geological time scale that separates the two species.

Other important invariant properties include the electrolyte-water composition of blood serum and many cells and tissues of phylogenetically related species in the adult state. Then, according to phase rule principles, the chemical potentials of water and electrolytes, as zero-order functions, remain constant for many species on the geological time scale that brings about the genetic distance among many of the first-order (adaptive) functions of distantly related species, as also among the closely related primates (man, apes, and monkeys). Genetic divergence can thus be measured both by anatomical standards at the organizing level, as well as by physicochemical standards at the molecular level.

The results of *King and Wilson* may be summarized by their statement that, in the comparison of man and chimpanzees, 'Their macromolecules are so alike that regulatory mutations may account for their biological differences.'

Pareto's General Sociology

Social systems as a whole conform to general principles of continuity ('synechism') as well as to laws of statistical probability, chance, and equilibrium. 'Synechism' (*Baldwin,* 1902; *Peirce,* 1892) is a word of Greek origin that signifies a property of continuity and a quality of being 'held together'. It applies to genetic continuity and invariance, as well as to principles of continuity of behavior with species. *Pareto*'s method, according to *Henderson* 'is an application of the logical method that has been found useful in all physical systems when complex situations involving many variables in a state of mutual dependence are described'.

Social systems must be studied according to the principles of applied anthropology rather than according to dualistic or mechanist principles that are ultimately behaviorist, or disconnected with value judgements. They can be understood only by methods previously applied to dynamic, thermodynamic, structured systems that are at the same time physiological and economic. Such systems comprise large numbers of interacting variables that are limited by certain general conditions of constraint.

In *Pareto*'s *General Sociology* (1926), certain fundamental human emotions are considered as elementary or fundamental. These include the sentiments, as related to such basic elements as the family, the home, patriotism, love of land and nature, national traditions and institutions and the like. Sentiments cannot be isolated, but are joined together synechistically in groups called 'aggregates'.

Pareto identifies many such aggregates, and relates them to what he calls 'derivatives'. Thus, the derivatives are related to the sentiments in which they originate. Thus, 'law' originates in the sentiments and aggregates of 'justice' or 'fair play', 'religion' originates in those of 'deity', the nature of the divine origin of things, and so on.

Two fixed laws apply to the derivatives. The first describes 'the persistence of aggregates'. In a modern nation, such as the United States, the first law applies to all sentiments and aggregates connected with permanent national institutions: the presidency, the constitution, the national anthem, and so on. These constitute permanent centripetal forces of synechism that contribute to invariance and conditions of constraint.

The second law refers to the 'residues of combinations'. This describes the possibilities of variations of social structure and functional conditions compatible with variations that do not conflict fundamentally with the sentiments, derivatives, and persistence of aggregates. Thus, there are strong analogies among all structural and organized systems — physicochemical, thermodynamic, biological, and social. 'Persistence of aggregates' corresponds to the zero-order functions or 'potentials'. Variations, evolution, and development depend on factors of chance or probability, and can occur under conditions of constraint imposed by the non-adaptive, non-evolving zero-order functions or potentials. All such systems must be adapted to a pluralistic rather than to a dualistic universe. However, internal states within any individual organism must also conform to monistic principles.

Chapter 12

Structure of Behavior

According to the principles of philosophical anthropology as described in chapter 11, all human behavior conforms within certain limits to the structural and functional principles that are accepted by the various societies and social orders that retain permanent features over long periods of time. It has been pointed out that any of the surviving folkways or mores must have some kind of functional value. Of course, certain venerable customs with no obviously useful functions may persist, but even so, it would be difficult to show that *no* function was served. The function may be simply one of preparing some bit of superstitious folklore, but this would merely turn out to be completely harmless: it would be classed as a mere idiosyncrasy or foible. It would be gratifying or amusing to human beings, and never too odious a nuisance in a well-ordered society governed by the 'pleasure principle'.

A well-ordered and structured society depends on well-ordered and structured behavior in all its members, including adults, children, and domestic animals. This presupposes reason and purpose in human laws and institutions and permanent standards of education, discipline, justice, and codes of ethics in all organized sections of the community. In modern societies in Europe and America, these principles derive from the ideas of the enlightenment, as formulated by *Locke* and *Hume* in England, *Rousseau, Voltaire* and the encyclopedists and philosophes in France, and the ideologists of constitutional democracy in the United States.

Well-ordered and structural behavior of each citizen in the United States is related to the structure of the government, as expressed by the three main branches of the civil departments: executive, legislative, and judicial. The presidential executive powers include the following divisions: legal, defense, agriculture, commerce, labor, communications (post office), interior (natural resources), foreign affairs, and so on. These spring from common needs found in all human orders, even at the most primitive levels: nutrition, defense, communication, reproduction, and shelter. Certain other functions related to the fine arts or to the theater, for example, have been more or less passed over in the United States in favor of the practical and applied arts, but institutions such as the Smithsonian (science), the National Gallery of Art, and various National Memorials maintain kinds of connections with the federal government. The

Congressional Library in Washington resembles in function the British Museum in London. Institutions such as these tend to structure and preserve the permanent forms of structure and behavior. The French Republic has always maintained permanent forms of theater to preserve the great classics of the language, and it maintains a Ministry of Fine Arts related to the Louvre and other great museums of Paris.

Thus, it is obvious that all great civilized nations and societies in modern history have tended to preserve traditional forms of behavior in all the recognized forms of structure and function, including military, law enforcement, and foreign relations. It is only in periods of barbarism or semi-barbarism that these standards tend to break down, and that human life tends to become chaotic, disorganized, nihilistic, and unstructured.

It has been the thesis of chapters 9 and 10 that well-structured human behavior depends in the last analysis on the evolution of human anatomy, morphology, and the continuity of human protoplasm and genes. These are the phylogenetic bases of well-ordered behavior and the foundations of structural, functional, and philosophical anthropology. Permanence and continuity of human behavior then depend on a principle called 'synechism' by *Peirce* (1878, 1892). This principle establishes permanent relations between structure, function, behavior, and survival. According to *Carnot*'s principle, it depends on the conservation of the zero-order thermodynamic functions (chemical potentials) and on the conservative biological functions (the given chromosomes, macromolecules, and protoplasm). The conservation and permanence of these *primaries* are the essential conditions for cultural spreading and diffusion of the *non-conservative* first-order functions of cultural anthropology.

Such variations are permissible under *Peirce*'s principle of 'tychism' (chance) (chapter 1). These principles, since the 19th century, have been related biologically to the 'struggle for existence'. This was identified (1905) as a struggle for 'negative entropy' (*Joseph,* 1973).

Biological Struggle

The second law of thermodynamics (principle of *Carnot-Clausius*) has been stated in the form 'the entropy of the *universe* tends toward a maximum'. This does not imply, as many biologists seem to have inferred, that the entropy of the *earth* tends always to increase. On the contrary, as *Schrodinger* has explained, the presence of great populations of living organisms, plant and animal in the biosphere of the earth depends on the retention and accumulation of cosmic amounts of negative entropy in the form of neuromuscular synthesis and the evolution of all kinds of living organisms, which are well-ordered, purposeful, and characterized by high rates of population growth and 'rates of living' (*Pearl,* 1928; *Joseph,* 1973).

Boltzmann (1905) explained biological entropy in the following way: 'The general struggle for existence of all living beings is not the struggle for the fundamental substances, for these fundamental substances, indispensable for all living creatures exist abundantly in the air, the water and the soil. The struggle is not a struggle for the energy, which in the form of heat, unfortunately not available, is present in a great quantity in every object, but it is a struggle for entropy, which is available when energy passes from the hot sun to the cold earth. In order to utilize in the best manner this passage, the plants spread under the rays of the sun the immense surface of their leaves, and cause the solar energy before reaching the temperature level of the earth to make syntheses of which as yet we have no idea in our laboratories. The products of the chemical kitchen are the object of the struggle in the external world.'

The accumulation of 'negative entropy' in the living world of plants and animals is explained as follows (*Joseph,* 1973). In their daily respiratory metabolism, animals produce carbon dioxide, water, and heat from nutrients such as carbohydrates, fats and proteins. For example in the combustion of 1 mole of glucose (180 g):

$$C_6H_{12}O_6 + 6\,O_2 = 6\,CO_2 + 6\,H_2O \tag{8}$$

$$\Delta H = -668.5 \text{ kcal,}$$
$$\Delta G = -690.5 \text{ kcal,}$$
$$T\Delta S = 22.0 \text{ kcal,}$$

and

$$\Delta G = \Delta H - T\Delta S.$$

Thus, carbon dioxide, water and heat are produced with an *increase* of entropy and an increase of cosmic disorder. However, the carbon dioxide and water are not lost to the biological or ecological process. They are returned or recycled in the systems of carbohydrates, such as glucose and starches, and become part of the living structure of all plants and animals. In the resynthesis of glucose, for example, $nh\nu$ calories of solar radiant energy are absorbed according to the reaction:

$$nh\nu + 6\,CO_2 + 6\,H_2O = C_6H_{12}O_6.$$

In this process, there is a decrease of entropy in which at the temperature of the earth:

$$T\Delta S = -22.5 \text{ kcal.}$$

Thus, in the combined processes of combustion and synthesis, + 22.5 kcal of radiant free energy are absorbed by the green leaves of plants in the process of photosynthesis (activated by chlorophyl) in the chloroplasts. This radiant energy is thus added to the chemical energy of living organisms in the form of carbohydrates (including cellulose and starches), and in the forms of other organic polymers. In the process of retaining this radiant energy, the plants withhold a vast quantity of entropy that otherwise would go into the *total* entropy of the universe. Thus:

Total entropy change = X + Y,

where X is the increase of entropy in the remainder of the universe, and where Y is the simultaneous entropy change of the biosphere.

Thus, the net increase of entropy is *less* than it would be if the earth were a dead planet, which retained no energy in the form of living organisms. This entails a large amount of entropy withheld from outer space. This can be referred to as 'negative entropy' in *Schrodinger*'s (1944) sense. The retention of negative entropy permits an increase of order in the biosphere, but this is no contradiction of *Carnot*'s principle, as many biologists seem to have inferred. It in no way implies any teleological or vitalistic conflict with the principles of chemical thermodynamics (*Joseph*, 1973).

The energy and 'negative entropy' accumulated by photosynthesis in the world of living plants can be rapidly transferred to the animal kingdom in the nutrition of herbivores and carnivores, such as animals and birds, and thereby transmitted to living cells, tissues, and protoplasm of all living species. This takes the form of a general competitive distribution of negative entropy among all living species. Thus, *Boltzmann*'s statement of the 19th century principle of the 'struggle for existence' can be expressed thermodynamically as a 'struggle for negative entropy'.

Thus, life depends on a general 'free for all' competitive struggle involving all living things, but it is mitigated by various forms of symbiosis or other forms of behavior related to mutual aid and cooperation. All forms of intra-tribal or international forms of structural, functional, and philosophical anthropology can be applied to mitigate the unfavorable or unpleasant aspects of the underlying competitive struggle for negative entropy.

Structure of Behavior

According to the principles of structural, functional, and philosophical anthropology (chapter 11), the structure of human behavior depends on the stabilization of human phylogeny and ontogeny or the conservation of all zero-order functions, and all conceivable adaptations of the first-order functions (anatomical, physiological, mental, and behavioral), and on the securing of adequate supplies of cosmic 'negative entropy'. Then in each human being at any age or state of development, behavior is constrained or limited by the morphological distribution of negative entropy, configurational free energy and dielectric energy in all the cells and tissues of the body. This determines irritability and responsiveness of each set of tissues in the neuromuscular system and all its divisions. It is related to the synthesis of the macromolecular polyelectrolytes, to the distribution of water and electrolytes, to the electrochemical or dielectric properties, and to resting and active metabolism.

The internal physiological and physicochemical systems tend to be invariant or univariant. Heart and circulating blood in the resting states tend to be limited by phase rule constraints in all active states. The accessibility or inaccessibility of any active or resting state is determined by *Carnot*'s principle, as stated in the form given in chapter 3. In this form, the second law may be stated for biological systems, including the human body, 'there are inaccessible states in the neighborhood of any given state'. A given state is always defined by the thermodynamic conditions of constraint: p, q, r, s, t, etc. These constitute a *set* of conditions, which will be denoted as S. When this set is fixed by the given special conditions, any other state, $S'' \dots S^D$, is *inaccessible*. Then according to *Carnot*'s principle, the given state in S is completely defined by the parameters p, q, r, s, t ... However, if any member of the set, p for example, is changed to a neighboring state, p', the initial state S becomes inaccessible, and S' becomes accessible. The same is true of any other inaccessible state in the neighborhood of S. This yields a definition of any given state, either normal or pathological. If any such state is defined by a set S' of parameters (p, q, r, s, t ...), the initial state becomes at least temporarily inaccessible.

Thus, any given normal or pathological process can be described as:

$$S \to S'.$$

A reversal of the process to the initial state is defined as:

$$S' \to S.$$

If the system is not completely reversible, the initial state may not be absolutely reversible or accessible. Thus, any relative state of reversibility would be defined by the set of parameters, p, q, r, s, t ... compared to the initial state S.

Thus, varying states of accessibility may be imagined or defined, in which any neighboring state becomes inaccessible to the given state. In human behavior, if the resting or inactive state is defined as S, then any given active state becomes accessible during physiological or behavioral activity. The *structure of behavior* is thus determined by the entire range of *neighboring states* accessible to each other and to S. The limits of behavior are thus determined by the limits of all possible or conceivable states of chemical morphology and metabolism (*Joseph*, 1973).

Hydration Energy

The dielectric properties of cells and tissues include the following: dielectric constant, D'', dielectric energy, configurational free energy and entropy, standard chemical potentials of the ions, and numerous other thermodynamic and electrochemical properties. All of these can theoretically be derived from the 'hydration energy' of any kind of inorganic ion; sodium, for example. In an aqueous solution at about 37 °C, the dielectric constant of water is about 80, and the theoretical value of the standard chemical potential of sodium, $\Delta\mu_{Na}{}^{\circ}$, is about -164 kcal/mole, referred to a vacuum, in which the value of the dielectric constant is 1.0. This follows from the equation of *Laidler and Pegis* (1957):

$$\Delta\mu_{Na}{}^{\circ} = \frac{N\, z_{Na}{}^2\, e^2}{2\, D''\, b_{Na}},$$

where N denotes *Avogadro*'s number, z_{Na} the charge of the sodium ion, taken as 1.0, e the electrostatic unit of charge, and b_{Na} the corrected ionic radius of sodium, 1.25 Å units.

In vacuo, the value of the dielectric constant is 1.0. Then the work of charging 1 mole of sodium vapor to 1 mole of sodium ions is calculated as 164 kcal when the above value of the corrected ionic radius is assumed. The value of 164 kcal is eight tenths the value of 205 kcal calculated for an ion with a radius of 1.0 Å unit.

Thus, *in vacuo* for an ion of 1.0 Å radius,

Molal work = $\Delta\mu_{Na}{}^{\circ}$ = 205 kcal.

In a solution of dielectric constant D'':

$$\mu_{Na}{}^{\circ} = \frac{205}{D''\, b_{Na}}.$$

In water, when $D'' = 80$, and $b_{Na} = 1.25$ Å,

$\mu_{Na}{}^{\circ} = 1.64$ kcal/mole.

Thus, the free energy or work of transferring 1 mole of sodium ions from an aqueous solution to a vacuum is:

W = $164 - 1.64 = 162.36$ kcal.

The molal work of hydration may be defined as the molal work of transferring sodium ions from an aqueous phase of dielectric constant 80 to a vapor phase in which the dielectric constant is 1.0. Let us assume that the ions are transferred instead from an intramuscular phase in which D'' is 30 to the vapor state. Then:

Molal work = $164 - 161.26 = 2.74$ kcal.

Hence it follows that the molal work of transferring sodium ions from an extracellular phase of the *milieu intérieur* can be obtained from the respective values of the free energy of hydration as referred to an intramuscular phase compared with the value for that of an aqueous extracellular phase of the *milieu intérieur*. Thus:

Molal work = $\Delta\mu_{Na}^\circ = 4.48 - 1.64 = 2.74$ kcal.

The function $\Delta\mu_{Na}^\circ$ has been defined in previous chapters as the change of standard chemical potential of sodium ions between an intracellular phase in its standard state as referred to an invariant *milieu intérieur*.

Thus, in the final analysis, the change of standard chemical of any ion can be referred to the difference in the free energies of hydration in each phase as referred to a theoretical vapor phase in which the dielectric constant is 1.0.

Configurational Free Energy

The change of standard chemical potential of sodium, denoted as $\Delta\mu_{Na}^\circ$, treated in the foregoing as the difference in free energies of hydration of sodium between two phases, has earlier been related to the dielectric energy of the intracellular phase (chapter 3) (*Joseph*, 1973).

$$c_{Na}''\Delta\mu_{Na}^\circ = RT\,[\Sigma c_i' - \Sigma(c_i)''],$$

where $\Sigma c_i'$ is the total ion concentration of blood plasma (about 0.315 mole/kg water), and $\Sigma(c_i)''$ is the total intracellular concentration of ions (bound plus free). The change of standard chemical potential $\Delta\mu_{Na}^\circ$ is related also to the action potential, E_a. Thus:

$$E_a = -\,96{,}500\,c_{Na}''\Delta\mu_{Na}^\circ \text{ (J)}$$

or

$$E_a = -\,23{,}060\,c_{Na}''\Delta\mu_{Na}^\circ \text{ (kcal)}$$

where E_a is expressed in volts, and $\Delta\mu_{Na}{}^\circ$ in kcal or joules. Accordingly,

$E_a = 43.4\ \Delta\mu_{Na}{}^\circ$ (mV),

where the change of standard chemical potential is expressed in kcal. Thus, taking the intramuscular values of $\Delta\mu_{Na}{}^\circ$ 2.74 kcal, as in the foregoing section, when D'' is 30, the calculated value of the action potential E_a becomes 118.8 mV, which is a fairly representative value for the action potentials of mammalian muscle (*Joseph*, 1973). When the intramuscular sodium concentration $c_{Na}{}''$ is taken as 0.028 mole/kg water, and $\Delta\mu_{Na}{}^\circ$ is 2.74 kcal/mole,

Dielectric energy = 0.028 × 2.74 = 76.7 cal/kg water.

$$\text{Work} = \frac{1}{4} \times 76.7,$$
$$= 19.2\ \text{cal},$$
$$= 82.4\ \text{J},$$
$$= 8.4\ \text{kg m}.$$

This value agrees to 5% with *Hill*'s value of 9.0 kg m for the work capacity of the arm muscles of an adult man (*Joseph*, 1973). Therefore, the work capacity can be calculated directly either from the action potential and sodium content, or from the total ionic content of skeletal muscle. It is therefore a dielectric property that is directly proportional to the change of the free energy of hydration, as measured by $\Delta\mu_{Na}{}^\circ$.

It can readily be inferred that any such neuromuscular behavioral process is directly related to corresponding changes of intracellular water, which can release free energy for the production of external work or for changes of isometric tension.

Intramuscular water is then part of a very labile state that can vary with respect to the dielectric constant, standard chemical potentials, and hydration energies of the ions. Therefore, all examples of neuromuscular behavior can be thought to depend on intracellular changes of the free energy of hydration, as expressed by *Born* (1920) and by *Laidler and Pegis* (1957). All such changes of state of intramuscular water involve increases of configurational entropy and free energy. When intracellular water passes from a well-ordered state of low dielectric constant (as in stretched muscle fibers) to a relative state of high dielectric constant (as in contracted muscle), there is a decrease in the free energy of hydration of the ions. This releases the same amount of free energy in the performance of external work (9 kg m in the human arm muscles). In the contracted state, the dielectric constant D'' approaches the value of 80 character-istic of the liquid state, which is one of lowered hydration energy. Thus, the muscular work depends on the change of configurational free energy of the stretched hydrated fibers, as compared to the contracted state in which the water approaches a state in which the dielectric properties approach those of the extracellular fluid.

The free energy of hydration may be defined as the molal work of transferring sodium ions from an aqueous phase of constant 80 to a vapor phase in which $\Delta\mu_{Na}°$ approximates 164 kcal. If the ions are transferred to the vapor phase from an intramuscular phase of dielectric constant 30, the calculated free energy of hydration in muscle is 4.38 kcal. Then the molal work of transferring to the vapor state is:

Molal work = 164 − 4.38 = 159.62 kcal.

In an extracellular fluid phase, in which the dielectric constant is 80:

Molal work = 164 − 1.64 = 162.36 kcal.

The change of standard chemical potential, $\Delta\mu_{Na}°$, is the difference in the two values of the free energies of hydration (muscle as compared with the extracellular fluid). This value is then:

$\Delta\mu_{Na}°$ = 4.38 − 1.64 = 162.36 − 159.62 = 2.74 kcal.

Thus, the change of standard chemical potential in the process is equal to the difference of the two values of the free energies of hydration (water versus muscle). This line of reasoning gives a physical meaning to the standard chemical potential of any ion in any phase by referring it to the work of transferring the given ion to the vapor state. This is then taken as the reference state for any kind of ion.

Relations between Tension and Length

Myofibrils may be treated according to the general thermodynamic relations between tension, length, and energy. In the general theory of elasticity:

dE = T dS + t dl,

where E denotes energy, S, the entropy, t represents tension, and length is denoted as l. T dS is related to thermal energy, and to the state of order or disorder. External work must be added to the system to increase the length at a given tension. When the independent variables are taken as T and t, rather than as S and l, the following result is obtained:

dG = − S dT + l dt,

where G is the *Gibbs* free energy.

From this thermodynamic equation, the following results have been obtained (*Joseph,* 1973):

$$l \, dt = - c_{Na}{}'' \, d\mu_{Na}{}^\circ.$$

The negative sign indicates that when l is constant (isometric contraction), the tension increases as $\mu_{Na}{}^\circ$ decreases. This corresponds to the fact that an increase of the dielectric constant corresponds to a decrease of dielectric energy, producing an increase of tension. Simultaneously, there is an increased rate of glycolysis in the altered state of water. The high energy of sodium ions is thus transferred to the contractile proteins after a transient period in which the hydrostatic pressure within the fibers is increased. For unit length and cross-sectional area, there is an integrated form:

$$t = 10.20 \, \bar{d}_w \times c_{Na}{}'' \, \Delta\mu_{Na}{}^\circ,$$

or

$$t = 8.6 \times \text{dielectric energy.}$$

In skeletal muscle, $c_{Na}{}''$ is about 0.03 mole/kg water, and $\mu_{Na}{}^\circ$ is about 2.8 kcal, or 11,712 J.
Then:

$$t = 8.6 \times 0.03 \times 11,172 = 3,022 \text{ g/cm}^2.$$

The tension, t, may also be calculated from the action potential by the conversion:

$$1 \text{ kcal} = 43.4 \text{ mV.}$$

Then:

$$t = 830 \, c_{Na}{}'' \, E_a.$$

When $c_{Na}{}''$ is taken as 0.03 mole/kg water, and the action potential E_a is 120 mV, then:

$$t = 3,000 \text{ g/cm}^2.$$

Accordingly, isometric tension and action potential are both related to hydration energy and dielectric energy. Thus, the following mechanical properties of muscle and other contractile tissues are related to the distribution of electrolytes and water as well as to the dielectric constant and hydration energy: length of myofibrils, the maximal work, and isometric tension. All of these properties would be highly labile and dependent on labile states of intracellular water, electrolytes, and tensile or contractile fibrous proteins. Thus, throughout the neuromuscular system, there exist numerous sets of contractile myofibrils in which dielectric energy and tension are in states of accessibility and inaccessibility, and in states of continuous and discontinuous activity. These processes depend on continuous changes of tension during which dielectric energy is transmitted from one set of structures to another.

Rates of intracellular glycolysis are also in continuous states of flux due to the secular fluctuations of dielectric constant and states of water (*Joseph*, 1973).

All such physicochemical and metabolic processes are intimately related to external behavior, such as changes of posture, external work, and speech or communication. Thus, in the effectors and efferent parts of the neuromuscular system, behavior is directly related not only to anatomical and morphological structure, but also to changes of physicochemical properties, as related mainly to hydration energies, electrochemical properties, and metabolism. These all depend on the limiting ranges of contractile states, which depend on *Carnot*'s principle as interpreted by *Caratheodory* (*Born*, 1948; *Joseph*, 1973).

Chapter 13

Synechism

The idea of 'synechism' may be illustrated by a motto to be found on certain coins issued by the government of the United States: *E Pluribus Unum* in the unification of many entities. It is a term derived from the Latin language, signifying a quality of being 'held together'. Thus, it can be applied to any unified continuum in which divergent elements are held together, organized or joined into a well-defined continuum or structure. *Peirce* contributed certain definitions to *Baldwin*'s (1902) *Dictionary of Philosophy and Psychology;* these included his definition of 'synechism', which follows.

'Synechism' (Gr. συνσγης), continuous holding together, from συν, εγσης), or to hold, not found in other languages. That tendency of philosophical thought that insists upon the idea of continuity as of prime importance in philosophy and in particular upon the necessity of hypotheses involving true continuity.

'A true *continuity* is something whose possibilities of determination no multitude of individuals can exhaust. Thus, no collection of points placed upon a truly continuous line can fill the line so as to leave no room for others, although that collection had a point for every value towards which numbers endlessly continued the decimal places could approximate nor if it contained a point for every possible permutation for all such values. It would be in the general spirit of synechism to hold that time ought to be supposed to be truly continuous in that sense.'

The purpose of any hypothesis is to render any otherwise inexplicable phenomena into the realm of things that are explicable. Thus, the practically continuous existence of the United States as a nation can only be explained by the reality of its organization as a synechistic unit held together by law, custom, human values, and common aggregates of sentiments (chapter 12).

In a similar way, the continuous existence in time of all the species of man *(Homo sapiens)* requires the concept of synechism to account for chronological development of morphology and behavior in historic and prehistoric epochs. This is true of all other species which, since their origins, have inhabited the various regions of the biosphere. Thus, the earth and its biosphere embrace a set of all actual and possible subsets, the coexistent loci of all habitats for all species. Just as time is considered in the foregoing as a true continuum, so must the same be true of geographical and atmospheric space. The earth consists of a synechistic unification of all the continents, rivers, seas, and oceans that evolve continuously in space and time. This is also true of all forms of life — plants as well as animals. Thus, true synechistic existence implies a unification and continuity of all biological species in a spatio-temporal continuum. This unification implies synechistic relationships that involve species, organisms, and all sets of environmental niches with all other parts of the universe on a cosmic time scale. Only relatively infinitesimal fragments of this practically infinite realm of space, time, and organism are accessible to experimental or laboratory observations in biology, psychology, or behavior. The rest requires foundations based on inductive inference, mathematics, definite laws of nature, and metaphysical inference based on principles such as synechism, reversibility, and continuity (*Joseph*, 1973).

The conservative or invariant zero-order functions are non-adaptive, and include the composition of blood plasma with respect to five components (water, $NaCl$, KCl, $CaCl_2$ and $MgCl_2$). Constant composition of blood plasma and other fluids of the *milieu intérieur* implies constant freezing points of the fluids and constant chemical potentials of each of the five components. This can be explained only by *Gibbs'* phase rule, which is based on the principle of *Carnot-Clausius*. Thermodynamic explanations are independent of mechanistic hypotheses and are free of the 'fallacy of misplaced concreteness' (*Whitehead*, 1925). The phase rule accounts for the continuous internal cohesion of the physicochemical systems of living organisms, including mammals and other vertebrates. Physiological homeostasis in general depends on principles of synechistic continuity.

Non-Mechanistic Behavior

Organistic behavior is distinguished from mechanistic behavior in that it always involves reversible and irreversible processes that occur in the cells and tissues of living organisms. It is based on the expenditure of stores of configurational free energy or 'negative entropy' in the neuromuscular system. The expenditure of free energy is lost to the external world, and becomes irreversible as a loss of heat. On a day-to-day basis, these losses are quantitatively replaced by a consumption of proteins and carbohydrates in the diet. These macromolecular substances are necessarily of biological origin, as are all the foods and nutrients consumed by human beings or by mammals in general. They originate in supplies of negative entropy produced in the green leaves of plants in the absorption of radiant photochemical energy derived from solar radiation. This appears to be the fundamental difference between non-mechanistic and mechanistic behavior.

The living mammalian or human organism attains its free energy and negative configurational entropy from biological materials. Typical man-made machines such as gasoline engines or railroad locomotives consume supplies of energy obtained from petroleum, coal, or other fossil fuels. These are completely unsuitable for the energy requirements of plants or animals without the aid of the photosynthetic process; oxidative combustion would yield carbon dioxide and water, necessary for conversion to glucose and starches, but this requires chlorophyll.

The digestion of fossil fluids or wood cannot occur in the mammalian organism. Man-made machines cannot obtain energy or entropy from biological material except under non-biological conditions, such as direct combustion at high temperatures (as in wood-burning heat engines). This distinction affords an absolute difference between mechanistic and non-mechanistic behavior. The latter always implies a living organism in which behavior is based on thermodynamic changes of state occurring in living protoplasm. The former is based on energy supplies which are not available to living organisms.

In living organisms, work and utilization of free energy depend on supplies of 'negative entropy' rather than on supplies of chemical bond energy (*Catchpole and Joseph,* 1974). In the living human being, for example, the exothermic heat of basal metabolism is lost to the body as heat or chemical bond energy. This heat is unavailable for external work (*Benedict and Cathcart,* 1913). Thus, in general:

$$\Delta G = \Delta H - T \Delta S,$$
$$\Delta G = \text{metabolic heat plus external work.}$$

When external work is performed by the activity of skeletal muscles of the human body, the overall efficiency is generally of the order of 10–30% (*Morehouse and Miller,* 1967). This is measured by the ratio:

$$\text{Efficiency} = \frac{T \Delta S}{\Delta H}.$$

Applying the same formula to the efficiency of isotonic, isothermal contraction of human or mammalian skeletal muscle, it is found that the efficiency of reversible contraction approaches 100% (*Catchpole and Joseph,* 1974). This requires that the contraction be reversible and isothermal, as taken over the entire cycle:

$$\int_1^1 dG = 0 \qquad \int_1^1 dH = 0 \qquad \int_1^1 dS = 0.$$
$$\text{(Relaxation)} \qquad\quad \text{(Contraction)} \qquad \text{(Relaxation)}$$

These are the conditions for invariance of physicochemical state over any conservative cycle (chapter 3). The negative balance of free energy and enthalpy, as measured by ΔG and ΔH, are at the expense of chemical bond energy resulting from the breakdown of glucose to lactic acid and the aerobic combustion of various metabolites (*Joseph*, 1973). These reactions are irreversible. This implies an entropic source of free energy rather than a source of chemical bond energy, such as adenosine triphosphate (*Catchpole and Joseph*, 1974).

Psychology: Introspectionist, Behaviorist, Gestalt

The introspectionist psychology of *William James* was based on a conceptual scheme that emphasized philosophical value judgements based on radical empiricism and philosophical pluralism. Various competing schools of experimental psychology criticized the subjective nature of introspection, as lacking an objective basis in experimental physiology, especially in the fields of the physiology of sensation and perception and in that of neuromuscular irritability and responses. In particular, behaviorist psychology, introduced by *J.B. Watson,* tended to seek a basis for human and animal behavior in nervous reflexes in various parts of the body, as they are affected by isolated stimuli of various kinds. The general tendency here was opposed to the subjectivity of introspection, which emphasized philosophical value judgements as important elements, at least in human behavior. For some perhaps obscure reasons, many so-called experimental psychologists have sought at all costs to eliminate value judgements from all the phenomenological sciences. This means in some cases to approach extreme forms of reductionism in an effort to reduce physiology to physics and chemistry and to mechanism.

At this point, it is pertinent to quote the point of view of *Claude Bernard* (chapter 9). 'He is not a physiologist who has not the organizing sense of that special coordination of the parts of the whole, characteristic of the vital phenomena. In the living being, things take place as though a certain "idea" stepped in which took into account the order in which the elements are grouped.'

This statement appears to show that by his general physiology and in his experimental medicine, *Bernard* fully appreciated the coordination of the parts of any biological organism to the whole, giving a definite 'sense' or 'idea' to all vital phenomena. This certainly shows that, in agreement with *Peirce*'s definition of 'firstness', *Bernard*'s views are synechistic or organistic rather than reductionist, mechanistic, or behaviorist.

Peirce's concept of 'objective idealism' is closely connected with *James*' 'radical empiricism' and 'philosophical pluralism'. In agreement with the thought of the 18th century enlightenment, *James*' pluralism was organized on the basis of phenomenological, non-mathematical observation of human values in psychology. This possibly accounts for its failure to attract many psychologists who opposed the introduction of conscious human values into experimental research. Here there seems to be a conflict with the theories and results of structural, functional, and philosophical anthropology, as presented in chapter 11.

Gestalt psychology, as developed in Europe by *Kohler, Koffka,* and *Wertheimer,* has a phenomenological basis common to other psychological disciplines.

Accordingly, the conceptual scheme of Gestalt psychology seems to be more in harmony with the 'organizing sense' of *Claude Bernard*'s general physiology and *Peirce*'s 'synechism' or 'holding together' than are the mechanist schemes of reductionist physiology.

When external work is performed by the activity of skeletal muscles of the human body, the overall efficiency is generally of the order of 10–30% (*Morehouse and Miller,* 1967).

Behavioral Values

According to the principles advanced in chapters 11 and 12, values form an essential group of sentiments, aggregates, and derivatives, related to perceptions that have arisen in various fields of functional, structural and philosophical anthropology. Thus, religious rites and many forms of literature, poetry, song and dance have arisen in the history of civilization. These are inseparable from many concurrent forms of esthetic and philosophical speculation. In terms of psychology, they are introspective rather than reductionist or geometrical.

One of the founders of Gestalt psychology, *Wolfgang Kohler,* who contributed to several of the experimental aspects of modern psychology, regarded the art of music as irreducible to physical or physiological acoustics. In this, he was in essential agreement with the views of *von Helmholtz,* who drew sharp distinctions between the art of music and the science of acoustics. *Sullivan* (1928) wrote on *Beethoven, His Spiritual Development,* in which the incommunicable values of spirituality and mysticism were sharply distinguished from the purely technical aspects of *Beethoven*'s art. To illustrate the aspects of Gestalt psychology that appear in both the art and science of music, the following considerations are advanced.

In the theory of harmony, an interval of the fifth is called the 'dominant' in any scale. Thus, on the keyboard of the modern pianoforte, the pitch of 'middle C' has a frequency of approximately 256 vibrations per second. The pitch of G in the scale of C approximates a frequency of 384 vibrations per second. The ratio of the two frequencies (dominant to tonic) is 3/2. This represents the dominant in any key. In the key of G, the dominant D vibrates in resonance to a frequency of 576 per second. This corresponds to a ratio of 3/2 referred to the tonic (384). The four strings of the violin are tuned to the keys of G, D, A, and E. The respective frequencies are 192, 288, 432, and 538. These correspond to the ratios of 3/2, 9/4, 27/8, and 81/16, as referred to the tonic C (128 vibrations per second). This law of musical intervals was known to Pythagoras among the ancient Greeks, who studied the acoustics of the monochord.

According to the principles of Gestalt psychology, the human ear responds to the interval of the fifth, or to the chord of the dominant as a whole; it does not necessarily distinguish the individual frequencies. In any key, the major triad would correspond to the chord C, E, G, or to 1, 3, and 5. In the key of G, the tones of the major triad are G, B, and D, also represented by relative frequencies of 1, 3, and 5. These chords in music are perceived by the musician and his auditors as 'gestalten' or 'configurations' rather than as the reductionist elements. Tonal perception in any auditor depends on the ability to perceive these relative intervals and chords in any key. In musical notation or symbolism, these 'gestalten' appear on the printed page as corresponding visual gestalten. The art of instrumental or vocal music depends on the technical skills required to read and perform many intricate 'gestalten' as they occur in unisons, harmony, and counterpoint to ensembles that range from unisons (as in *Bach*'s unaccompanied violin or cello sonatas) to ensembles of varying complexity. These embrace all forms of chamber music (trios, quintets, and the like) up to works for full orchestra or for choral music on the scale of oratorios or opera.

The values in music or any of the related arts depend on principles of Gestalt psychology, sensory perceptions and esthetic behavior. At any level beyond that of an absolute beginner or novice, the values are irreducible to behaviorist skills or to pure introspection. At higher levels of performance, the art of music may be integrated with the arts of ballet, tragedy, comedy, religious ritual, or theatrical spectacle. These may engage the talents of scores of instrumentalists, vocalists, and dancers, as well as the skills of costume designers, the choreographers, chorus and orchestra directors, and even in certain operas the skills of horses, camels, and elephants. In any but the rarest of cases, these intricate 'gestalten' represent value judgements that are all but inaccessible to the philosopher, the behaviorist or to the introspective psychologist. They are also irreducible to reductionist or mechanistic physiology. It was acknowledged by *von Helmholtz* (1862/1954) that the art of music was practically irreducible to the sciences of physical or physiological acoustics. In general, with practically no exceptions, biological scientists have lacked the 'organizing sense' that is required for the creation of great works requiring the collaboration of the dramatist, composer, and librettist. This requires an instinctive 'synechism' or unification, as exemplified by the ancient principle of the dramatic unities. Thus, the characters in great drama are 'held together' by a plot in which action, language, and character are continuous or inseparable in the sense of a true continuum or synechistic organization. In certain forms of music, the structure is 'held together' by instrumental parts, known as the 'continuo'. Because of ancient habits of Cartesian and Newtonian reductionism, it has appeared to many others (non-scientists) that scientists are in danger of losing the 'organizing sense' or sense of pluralistic 'gestalten' that are the essence of significant values in all the fine arts. From the point of view of metaphysics or philosophical anthropology, all permanent values depend on a true synechistic continuum that unifies all the isolable individual elements or units.

Emergent Evolution

The general principle of synechism (*E Pluribus Unum*) can be applied not only to all anthropological or social groupings of human beings at any level of complexity, but also to all groups within any *biocoenose*. This term, as used by *Wheeler* (1928), includes 'communities of plants and animals of many species living in particular environments, such as swamps, deserts, rain forests, etc. ... veritable welters of organisms of many species, all interacting with one another in complex predatory, parasitic, and symbiotic relationships, but forming wholes in which the experimental field naturalists can readily distinguish general adaptive patterns ...' We may truthfully say that there is not on the planet a single animal or plant that does not live as a member of some biocoenose.

The principle of emergent evolution, as related to that of synechism and philosophical pluralism, is of general applicability and finds illustrative examples in the world of organic substances that form homologous series, as well as in biology.

Among American and British biologists and philosophers committed to the general synechistic principles of emergent evolution, the following may be included: *Alexander, Gordon, Holt, Jennings, Morgan, Ogden, Parker, Sellars,* and *Spaulding* (*Wheeler*, 1928). The common set of beliefs of this group can be summarized in the words of *Spaulding:* 'Certain specific relations organize parts into wholes ... certain states of affairs are identical with new properties and are different and distinct from the individual parts and their properties. Therefore, the *reduction* of these new properties to those of the parts in the *sense of identification* and the finding of a *causal determination* also in the same sense is *impossible*.'

The matter has been stated in the following way by *Willstatter* (1929): 'Until now it was taken for granted in chemistry that the properties of components in chemical compounds disappear, but that in mixtures of substances they are retained. This is an antiquated viewpoint ... Mixtures may actually possess the nature of new chemical compounds.' *Willstatter*'s opinion confirms that of

Spaulding that the reduction of the properties of protoplasm to those of its constituent components is *impossible.*

'... This compels us, in considering the evolution of organic substances to rely not upon those alterations in which this or another isolated compound may be subjected, but to bear in mind alterations which take place in complex mixtures of organic substances' (*Oparin,* 1938).

These views of an eminent biochemist and of a prominent biologist emphasize an organicist point of view, which regards protoplasm as a synechistic continuum that depends on its phylogenetic development in cosmic space and time, rather than on distinct isolable and identifiable principles of causality and sufficient reason. The properties of protoplasm arise as emergent entities that originate in primitive antecedents.

Organicist views were also held by *Henderson* (1928), as also by *Bernard* (1878) in their respective treatments of blood plasma and the *milieu intérieur* as invariant continua, developing synechistically from antecedent biological and environmental fluids (sea water) that contained water and the five physiological ions of Ringer solution (sodium, potassium, calcium, magnesium, and chloride). Thus, mammalian blood is an emergent biological fluid that cannot be resolved, reduced, or understood entirely with reference to its isolable components: water, electrolytes, hemoglobin, and other intracellular colloids, serum albumins, globulins, and various kinds of purified isolable components. Its functions as a biological system depend on its organicist character, as expressed by *Carnot*'s principle, by *Gibbs*' 'equilibrium of heterogeneous substances', and by *Bernard*'s principle of an invariant *milieu intérieur* (*Joseph,* 1973). Biological continuity and synechism require the conservation of all first-order thermodynamic functions or potentials, and the conservation of invariant genetic properties related to phylogeny and speciation.

Thus, the continuous and permanently invariant properties of all biological systems are to be regarded as synechistic with phylogeny and ontogeny, but also with biological behavior, which is always constrained and restricted by the nature of chemical morphology and organicism. This principle is comprehensible only on the basis of *Carnot*'s principle, as applied to the nature of protoplasm, as maintained by continuous supplies of cosmic 'negative entropy' (*Joseph,* 1973). It cannot be derived from mechanistic principles, as they are applied to inorganic or non-protoplasmic systems, which derive energy and entropy from non-biological sources, as in man-made heat engines that operate on fossil fuels, electrical energy, or other non-biological supplies, inaccessible as materials for living plants or animals.

Since all living systems depend ultimately on solar radiance as sources of energy and 'negative entropy', all life in the biosphere is synechistic with the cosmic origin of the earth and solar system. It depends therefore on the permanence of the laws of cosmology as applied to the sun, the earth, and the entire solar system, as they have developed and continue to develop as synechistic continua that persist in cosmic space and time. This line of thought is given expression by *Carnot*'s principle in modern science and by *Parmenides*' principle in ancient philosophy (chapter 3).

Phase Rule Conditions of Synechism

In any multicellular organism, such as mammals or birds (*vie constante*), synechistic and organistic unity is maintained by phase rule conditions of invariance and constraint (*Joseph*, 1971a, b; 1973). Any such heterogeneous system consists of a large number of intracellular and extracellular phases, including blood plasma, hemolymph, and other extracellular fluids. All such phases contain water distributed as a component among p coexistent distinct phases. According to phase rule conditions of invariance (*Gibbs*, 1875, equation 77):

$$\mu_{H_2O}{}' = \mu_{H_2O}{}'' \dots = \mu_{H_2O}{}^p.$$

Thus, the chemical potential of water, μ_{H_2O}, is constant throughout a system of p phases in the physiological or thermodynamic standard state of invariance. This represents a resting state in which all exchange processes of five components (H_2O, $NaCl$, KCl, $CaCl_2$, $MgCl_2$) are reversible and isothermal. This represents a standard state, with reference to which all neighboring states are inaccessible or *secondary*.

Thus, all intracellular and extracellular phases are related to fixed conditions of thermodynamic state (*Carnot*'s principle), which makes possible a true synechistic distribution of the water and inorganic ions throughout the organism. The actual distribution of water and ions is determined by the standard value of δ for the system and by the values of $\Delta\mu_i{}^\circ$ for the various ions (*Joseph*, 1973). Thus, the actual distribution of water and electrolytes is determined by the dielectric properties (hydration energies), by the acid-base balance in each type of structure, and by the standard invariant properties of the *milieu intérieur*. The dielectric properties and the acid-base balance tend to be functions of one variable, the chemical morphology of the emergent properties of protoplasm or the extracellular colloids in any phase. Since this system is a function of the age, growth, and development, it may be regarded as a univariant property in a system with one degree of freedom, in which μ_{H_2O}, μ_{NaCl}, μ_{KCl}, μ_{CaCl_2}, and μ_{MgCl_2} are invariant in blood plasma and other extracellular fluids.

Thus, the entire physicochemical system is 'held together' by phase rule conditions of reversible distribution, and *Carnot*'s principles of invariance and constraint. These determine the chemical morphology in any tissue or set of tissues at any point on the standard curve of growth and development.

In such a heterogeneous system in its standard state, four other phase rule conditions of reversible distribution are applicable, describing the distributions of the four electrolyte components:

$$\mu_{AB}' = \mu_{AB}'' \cdots = \mu_{AB}^{p},$$

. . . .
. . . .

$$\mu_{AB_2}' = \mu_{AB_2}'' \cdots = \mu_{AB_2}^{p},$$

where μ_{AB}' and μ_{AB_2}' refer to the chemical potentials of the two kinds of electrolytes — binary and ternary. Type AB refers to binary electrolytes such as NaCi and KCl, whereas type AB$_2$ refers mainly to $CaCl_2$ and $MgCl_2$. Accordingly, electrolyte distribution satisfies conditions of the form:

$$\Delta\mu_{Na} = \Delta\mu_{K} = \frac{1}{2}\Delta\mu_{Ca} = \frac{1}{2}\Delta\mu_{Mg} = -\Delta\mu_{Cl} = \delta,$$

where δ denotes the equivalent change of chemical potential. Hence, in the standard resting state of invariance:

$$\Delta\mu_{Na} = \Delta\mu_{Na}° + RT \ln \frac{c_{Na}''}{c_{Na}'}.$$

Since in the normal resting state, $\Delta\mu_{Na}$, c_{Na}'', and c_{Na}' may be treated as constants, the change of standard chemical potential, $\Delta\mu_{Na}°$, may also be regarded as a constant that depends on the dielectric constant of each phase and on the free energies of hydration.

The synechistic quality of being held together in space and time establishes the unity of any organism, such as any given human being, as a well-ordered individual over a time scale that extends from birth to normal senescence. Since human behavior is synechistic, 'held together', and continuous with anatomy and morphology, it is also a time-dependent well-ordered entity that depends on the principles of *Carnot* and *Gibbs,* and on the principles of constraint that were described by *Bernard* (1878).

Human or animal behavior can be possibly described by purely physico-chemical and physiological parameters that refer to processes in the sensory and motor nerves and in other parts of the neuromuscular systems. All such processes seem to involve reversible cyclic or oscillatory changes of dielectric constant, dielectric energy, and hydration energies of intracellular and extra-cellular water and ions. Thus, all observable neuromuscular behavior appears to depend on highly integrated processes that involve well-ordered protoplasmic states of water. These processes are generally continuous, isothermal, labile, and reversible, involving always certain well-defined normal states that become temporarily accessible. Thus, all complex behavioral processes involve large numbers of actual or possible states, and a temporal succession of hydration energies that are locally reversible, but which may involve large outputs of exothermic metabolic energy. Thus, metabolism tends to fluctuate with behavior, according to the fluctuations of intracellular water and hydration energies. One of the functions of intracellular glycolytic metabolism is to transfer 'negative entropy' from nutrient sources of glucose to macromolecular substances, thus maintaining states of low entropy, molecular order, and synechism. This must be considered to be one of the many examples of fundamental biological behavior in the facility of organizing relatively disordered external relations into highly organized internal perceptions and *a postiori* experiences. Thus, in growing children, assimilated experience, understanding and knowledge would seem to depend on an organized principle of reordering relatively disordered external phenomena into well-organized neuromuscular behavior, voluntarism, and value judgements. The more highly the development of will and idea is attained in the adult human being, the greater is the accumulation of highly ordered 'negative entropy', acting as an organizing faculty.

This impression of the nature of integrative emergent factors would then appear to agree with the criteria given by *Claude Bernard* regarding the organizing faculty found in all living things (chapter 8). The principle depends on chemical morphology, considered not only on the basis of macroscopic analysis, but also on that of physicochemical state and structure. Negative entropy is related to the hydration energy of the ions in any structure, as determined by the state of intracellular water.

Human Creativity

According to the second law of thermodynamics (*Carnot*'s principle), all closed or isolated physicochemical systems tend to approach states of equilibrium at rates that depend on special conditions. Such systems include biological organisms in which equilibrium and steady state conditions may be maintained for many years, as in the aging processes of human beings and other mammals. Essentially, as *Schrodinger* (1944) has shown, this depends on nutritional supplies of 'negative entropy', which depend indirectly on conversion of radiant solar energy or negative entropy by chloroplasts in the green leaves of plants. In the form of glucose, starches, and other carbohydrates, the products of photosynthesis are consumed in animal nutrition, and remain as sources of configurational free energy in all cells and tissues of the mammalian body (*Joseph,* 1973).

This leads to the following scheme for transfer of entropy to the external world:

	Organism	Environment	Process
I.	Increase of entropy	decrease of entropy	creative increase of order
II.	Increase of entropy	increase of entropy	destructive increase of disorder
	Increased rate of metabolism, compensated by nutrition and assimilation of negative entropy		
III.	Decrease of entropy	increase of entropy	reversal of steps I and II within the organism; maintenance of steady state

According to this scheme, constructive human creativity by the human organism requires a transfer of negative entropy to a meaningful increase of order in the external world. To maintain internal order in the organism, a supply of negative entropy in the form of biological nutrients is required. The ultimate source of negative entropy is the constant supply of solar radiant energy, available for photosynthesis. Thus:

Sunlight → photosynthesis → nutrients → animal morphology
Animal morphology → free energy → purposeful creativity.

Thus, the ultimate source of human creativity is to be sought in the constant and continuous supply of protoplasmic free energy in the sun.

Relatively permanent supplies of configurational free energy are available to maintain irritability, tension, and responsiveness throughout the animal organism. This free energy is distributed in such a way as to determine all the permutations of accessible states in the body. Thus, the range of all possible redistributions among the coordinated secondary states. The distributions and redistributions correspond to one-to-one biunivocal intracellular states of water, hydration energies, chemical potentials, metabolic rates, and types of glycolytic, proteolytic, and lipolytic metabolism. Thus, all animal and human behavior depends ultimately on the distribution of configurational free energy and negative entropy in the organism. This corresponds to maximal free energy, minimal entropy, and basal metabolic rates in the resting state, and to states of relative disorder, increased disorder with increases of metabolic rates in active states of production of heat, work, or isometric tension.

Free energy or negative entropy is available for transfer to the external world either for constructive tasks (increase of order) or for the purposes of destruction (increases of disorder).

This is either dissipated as heat, cosmic disorder, or destructive activities, or it is employed constructively in various kinds of creative processes. The latter would include all significant endeavors in the sciences, technologies, the arts and letters, and in the solution of the various problems that arise in human societies.

As an illustration of the principle of order and disorder in human activities, let us consider the problem of correct spelling and sentence structure in human language and communication. If we consider the proper spelling of the word 'entropy', we find six different alphabetical letters ordered in only one appropriate way. Thus, there is only one correct spelling of the word. Any other ordering of the six letters results in a misspelled word. This is intolerable in purposeful well-ordered communication. As compared with one acceptable arrangement of the six letters, it will be found that there are 719 possible ways of misspelling entropy, as by random selection of the six letters subject to pure chance. The total number of ways of ordering six different objects according to chance is:

$$W = 6! = 6 \times 5 \times 4 \times 3 \times 2 \times 1 = 720.$$

Thus, out of 720 possible arrangements, only one is correct. According to a standard formula for entropy:

$$S = k \ln P,$$

where S denotes entropy, and P denotes the probability of any state of order or disorder. The lower limit corresponds to the value $S = 0$, and $P = 1.0$, which imply perfect ordering in a system.

A negative value of S implies a low probability of randomly selecting the six letters in 'entropy' is:

$$P = 1/720,$$

where 720 is the total number of possibilities. Therefore:

$$S = - k \ln 720.$$

In the word 'entropic' there are seven letters to be arranged in one correct order. Therefore:

$$S = - k \ln 7! = - k \ln 5,040.$$

As a general formula, we find:

$$P = \exp (- S/k).$$

Thus, the *a priori* probability of any given set of permutations decreases exponentially with the entropy. The maintenance of a state of *negative entropy* in living cells and tissues implies a stabilization of a degree of order that is conceivable only in living systems based on protoplasmic structures. This must be based on a multiplicity of well-ordered and structured phases in a heterogeneous physicochemical system.

Lability of Protoplasm

Whereas there is only one correct way to spell any word such as entropy or energy, there may be many possible ways of structuring a sentence to express a given thought. The exact form chosen by a given writer depends not only on the exact thought that he wishes to express, but also on the reader or group of readers to whom he addresses himself. In any case, the choice may be very complex, and may be based on quite arbitrary purposes: to convey information, perceptions, conceptions, or insights with maximum economy, a minimum of effort, and a maximum of pleasurable communication. The perfect sentence or paragraph is ordered in such a way as to represent a state of low entropy or very low probability *(a priori)*. The ability of a writer to achieve perfect expression of any line of thought is therefore a measure of his ability to convey internal states of negative entropy to the written page, or to spoken language.

Thought, as expressed in any form, then represents very free and labile forms of rearrangements of entropy. According to the general concept of synechism as an organized 'holding together', it tends to unify speaker and auditor, and to transfer negative entropy from one to the other. The concept of verbal or spoken fluency therefore implies very labile states of protoplasm in the neuromuscular and auditory neurones and receptors of all parties to human communication and discourse. The arts of communication thus depend on the lability of protoplasmic entropy or energies of intracellular hydration and molecular structure.

Chapter 14

Reason

If, as stated by *Whitehead* (1929), the function of reason is to promote the art of life, there can be no better formulation of this principle than that contained in the Declaration of Independence, threefold human rights to 'life, liberty, and the pursuit of happiness'. This derives from the main principles of English empiricism, as stated in the 18th century enlightenment, according to the anthropocentric views of *Locke, Hume,* and *Alexander Pope*. In the early years of the 20th century, *William James* expressed similar views in *Radical Empiricism* and *A Pluralistic Universe*. Also in agreement with this point of view was the special form of objective idealism, as developed by *Peirce* in the late decades of the 19th century.

In a group of essays entitled *Chance, Love and Logic, Peirce* outlined the basis of a metaphysical treatment of human reason, based on a threefold basis of evolutionary change. In this scheme, chance is expressed by the term derived from the Greek word 'tychism'. Logic, or the principle of being coherently 'held together' is expressed as 'synechism', as explained in chapter 13. Thirdly, 'the pursuit of happiness' could be expressed by the term 'agapism', derived from the Greek word 'agape' which includes all forms of human creative or evolutionary love, expressed in the broadest possible sense.

Peirce's choice of the principles of chance, love, and logic bears a striking resemblance to the triadic principles of 1776. *Peirce* used terms adapted from the Greek language to represent the three principles, i.e.:

Chance = 'tychism' (Gr.) = Liberty (1776),
Love = 'agapism' (Gr.) = Pursuit of happiness (1776),
Logic = 'synechism' (Gr.) = Life (continuity and order of life (1776).

The relation of life to reason depends on a synechistic quality of life being 'held together' in a continuum that includes fundamental qualities of *reason*, i.e. liberty (tychism) and happiness (agapism). Thus, *Whitehead*'s fundamental definition of 'reason' is deeply related to the principles of 1776, and to the rational empiricism of *Locke, Hume, Peirce,* and *James* (chapters 4 and 8).

Agapism (Evolutionary Love)

In the triadic relationship outlined above, 'life' may be described by a quality of 'firstness' that should be attributed to protoplasm. No form of life that is known to science can exist in any but a protoplasmic state. Feelings, sensations, and emotions are familiar aspects of 'agapism'. Experience teaches us to attribute them to all living men, women, and children. Such feelings are characterized by the quality of 'secondness', because we experience them only in relation to labile forms of protoplasm. We do not attribute feelings to inanimate objects such as furniture and automobiles. The experiences of life include agapistic feelings not only between subjects of protoplasmic origin (firstness), but also those which embrace reactions toward inanimate objects. If these relations are permanently ordered, 'held together', continuous and synechistic, they would be invariant in time. This is the principle of 'tychism', or evolution by fortuitous change. The external physical world operates not only by principles of immutable law (such as gravitation, mechanical necessity, electromagnetism, and thermodynamics), but also it is subject to what has generally been experienced as uncontrollable chance (hurricanes, floods, blizzards, and other unpredictable meteorological conditions). Chance operates in other ways to affect human life: illness, mortality, accidents, and many kinds of unpredictable fortuitous events.

The element of liberty or freedom depends on permutations and combinations that arise in the lives of nations and individuals, resulting from the operations of tychism. Thus, in *Pareto*'s general sociology, synechistic order is maintained by his principle of the 'persistence of aggregates', including all sentiments and groups of sentiments or residues (chapter 11). However, societies develop through a principle known as the 'residues of combinations'. Due to the operation of random and fortuitous chance, certain of the residues can change within new permissible limits which arise through the laws of probability.

Accordingly, human reason can develop according to the principles of evolution conforming to synechism, agapism, and tychism:

I. Synechism	firstness	protoplasm	life
II. Tychism	secondness due to fortuitous change	lability of protoplasm	life
III. Agapism	thirdness	ordering of I and II	reason

It appears then that reason is an emergent property of life related to the evolution of agapism from labile protoplasm. We thus arrive at a definition of reason as the 'promotion of the pursuit of happiness'. *Whitehead* (1929) has previously defined the function of reason as being 'to promote the art of living'. There is no reason to distinguish the 'pursuit of happiness' from the 'art of living'.

Thus, the principles of 1776 directly relate 'life, liberty, and the pursuit of happiness' to the same principles of purposeful evolution described as 'chance, love, and logic' or as 'tychism, agapism, and synechism'. Laws of chance and logic operate everywhere in the universe of physics, chemistry, and mathematics. They also operate in the universe of biology, but the element of agapism or the 'pursuit of happiness' cannot really be explained if one is not to arrive at a soulless universe devoid of all value. Reason is inconceivable without the principle of human happiness and values.

Thirdness

Three modes of evolution have been mentioned as operative in the world, and have been discussed by biologists and philosophers over a period of more than a century. These include Darwinian natural selection, or evolution by fortuitous chance. This has seemed to many to lack any ordered purposefulness or directedness, and has found no uniformity of agreement. A second principle, described by *Peirce* (1892) as 'anancism' is a doctrine of evolution by mechanical necessity in which any stage of the process at any time leads necessarily to the following series of steps. Development can then be described as a synechistic continuity, which is predetermined to certain goals by a kind of 'predetermined harmony' earlier described by *Leibniz* by means of his principle of sufficient reason. A third principle is creative love, and this has been advocated by philosophers such as *Henry Adams,* interested mainly in the philosophy of history. Especially in *Mount St. Michel and Chartres, Adams* considered the evolution of art, architecture, and religion in medieval Europe from the synechistic point of view, the quality of being 'bound together' of all aspects of national life. The emphasis was definitely on the role of creative love in the creation of medieval ways of life (*Adams,* 1900).

The word *agape* derived from the Greek αγαπε (love, love feast) was applied in early religious forms to denote a general principle of love, bearing on human relations embracing all men, women, and children, forms of friendship or brotherly love, and the love of religious deities. In ancient Greek cultures, agapism was related to the god Eros and to the goddess Venus.

In the great poem *On the Nature of Things,* the poet *Lucretius* addressed himself to Venus in the following way: 'Mother of Aeneas and his race, delight of man and gods, life-giving Venus, it is your doing that under the wheeling constellations of the sky all nature teems with life, both the sea that buoys up our ships and the earth that yields our food. Through you all living creatures are conceived and come forth to look upon the light.' This theme is continued throughout the poem. It is clear that in this poem the Lucretian theme of the creative power of love differed as greatly as possible from the blind tychistic Darwinian power of natural selection or evolution by fortuitous chance.

In a similar way, it differed greatly from what *Peirce* was later to call 'anancism' or evolution by mechanical necessity. The fundamental distinction between *Peirce*'s 'anancism' and all forms of 'agapism' or evolutionary love was clearly seen by *Adams* (1900) in his autobiographical work *The Education of Henry Adams.*

The Dynamo

The essential distinction between agapism and anancism was perceived and elucidated in a well-known chapter *The Dynamo and the Virgin.* Greatly impressed by an Exposition of Mechanical Science held at about the turn of the century, *Adams* was led to serious reflections concerning the motive force that provided the tremendous spiritual energy necessary for the creation of the great cathedrals of the Middle Ages and of the religious art of the renaissance. This spiritual energy, as expressed in the agapistic love of Venus, the Virgin and the Madonna, was the living force of that period of history. This found expression not only in the paintings of *Leonardo, Raphael, Titian,* and *Giorgione,* but also in the sculpture and architecture of *Michelangelo* and in the 17th century Flemish art of *Rubens.* After this last great outburst of passion in Flanders, the art of painting seemed to lose much of the energy derived from Venus, the Virgin and from Eros.

As *Adams* was to write in the year 1900, 'Symbol or energy, the Virgin had acted as the greatest force in the Western world ever felt, and had drawn men's activities to herself more strongly than any other power, natural or supernatural, had ever done; the historian's business was to follow the track of the energy; to find where it came from and where it went to; its complex sources and shifting channels; its values, equivalents, conversions.'

Thus, comparing this force with that of the 20th century dynamo, 'All the steam in the world could not, like the Virgin, build Chartres.' By the year 1900, the power of the Virgin and of Venus had become so attenuated, particularly in America, that the power of the steam engine, the gasoline engine, and of the hydroelectric dynamo became unchallengeable by Eros and Venus. The entire character of the age became dominated by the spirit of anancism or evolution by mechanical necessity. By the middle of the 20th century, sources of nuclear energy had been tapped. This is on a cosmic scale and completely submerges the feeble energies available to mankind on the basis of a meager 3 or 4 kcal/day, obtainable from nutrient sources. Thus, the principle of agapism or the pursuit of happiness on the human scale is clearly challenged by the principle of anancism based on cosmic sources of energy.

Reason

There are three functions of reason: to live, to live well, and to live better (*Whitehead*, 1929). Few will be found to object to this proposition. The obvious scientific criticism would refer to the subjectivity of the adverbs 'well' and 'better'. These clearly depend on the subjective tastes and values of each person. Individual tastes depend on so many unpredictable and undefinable peculiarities that they can be measured only by statistical rather than by absolute standards. Hence the concept of reason itself has an element of ambiguity that is ultimately tychistic – hence a matter of chance, probability, and entropy.

Thus, in art and literature, the concepts of classical, baroque, romantic, and popular can never be subject to permanent criteria that can satisfy all who have some claim to lives of reason or human values. Particularly this is true when it is a matter of values or relevance of the ancient classics. Experience shows that these works lose value or relevance when the reader can find no meaningful or pleasurable reference to his own conditions of life. Thus, for the most part, reasonable values apply mainly to the present and to material of the contemporary world. Here it is safe to refer the pursuit of happiness to each individual, and to apply the ancient adage – 'do no harm'.

It has been found in earlier chapters that the principles of rational empiricism tend to generate a preference for pluralism rather than for any strict form of absolutism or 'thin' abstractions. This tends toward broad tolerance and catholicity of taste rather than to any form of intolerant pedantry. Here the tendency is for synechistic agapism, and for various kinds of tychistic nonconformism. That the element of chance and unrestricted tolerance can never be absent should be taken for granted in all historical and geographical regions of space time. This follows from the known principles of philosophical anthropology, which accept the maxims of *Pope* and of *Plotinus* (chapter 11).

It would follow from this line of thought that reason, measured as the pursuit of happiness should be based on a science of organicism and biologically structured behavior. This would be based on *William James'* radical empiricism, philosophical pluralism, and on the concepts of Gestalt psychology rather than on those of experimental behaviorist psychology. Organicist conceptions, insofar as they can be reduced to science, can be based only on *Carnot*'s principle and *Gibbs'* phase rule, as applied to the structure and behavior of living protoplasm. They cannot be based on strictly mechanistic conceptions which lack the 'sense of organization' found only in the properties of protoplasm based on labile states of water and hydration energies.

Antirationalism

Science is based on human reason, and can be considered to be completely compatible with *Peirce*'s concept of 'objective idealism'; it is attainable only by a process of detachment of each individual scientist from his own egoistic tendencies to wish fulfillment or fantasy. This demands a kind of selflessness not usually attainable by many men. Many individuals, who have never quite attained the level of objective detachment required for the pursuit of science in physics and chemistry, have acquired sufficient intellectual qualifications to criticize scientific technology on the basis of its alleged indifference to human values in general.

In modern times, the rationalist attacks on certain aspects of applied science or technology would be exemplified at its best by such men as *Bertrand Russell, Albert Einstein,* and *A.N. Whitehead.* The irrational antiscientific attitude would perhaps be best represented by such writers as *D.H. Lawrence,* who seem to have been opposed to the claims of pure thought. The empiricism of *Locke* and *Hume* would not have excluded agapism as an important ingredient in the life of reason or the pursuit of happiness. Neither would it have explained pure objective thought in a synechistic 'holding together' of all the sciences, intellectual disciplines, technologies, and the various fine arts, including *belles lettres.*

There is no doubt that an attitude of introspective subjectivism has important claims in the pursuit of happiness. This is the attitude of pure agapism or evolutionary love, which means devotion to the ancient love of the gods. However, as pointed out in earlier paragraphs, this can lead to a mystique of antirationalism which in certain cases produces a common kind of antiscientific bias found in some intellectuals. This can be balanced only by a just estimate of 'man's place in nature', in which due consideration is given to the 'fitness of the environment', where this refers not only to the immediate geophysical and geochemical conditions, but also to those of cosmic space and time.

Such a view does justice to the agapistic and emotional nature of the fully developed human being, as in philosophical anthropology (chapter 11), but would resist any attempt to reduce human life to the dimensions of behaviorist or reflex psychology, presumably limited to the principles of simple location of atoms and molecules in the Cartesian or Newtonian sense. The dimensions of the problem may be referred only to the empiricism of the 18th century enlightenment, as understood by *Locke* and *Hume,* qualified by their species of skeptical humanism. It cannot be reduced to the principles of pure chance and logic, the basic point of view of modern experimental physicochemical science.

Much of the antirationalism of recent years can be attributed to the agapistic indifference of physicochemical thought as it has been based on the post-Cartesian and post-Newtonian applications of chance and logic. This has led to mechanist concepts in biology and to behaviorist notions in psychology and education. It has also led to positivistic rejections of *Alexander*'s metaphysics of 'natural piety' (*Collingwood*, 1938). *Goethe*'s rejection of the Newtonian theories of light and color vision was based on the difficulty or impossibility of reducing the natural spectrum of white light to the very wide range of colors observed in nature or imitated on the palette of the painter.

Structure, Function, and Change

The qualities of structure, function, and directed change may be designated respectively as firstness, secondness, and thirdness. Firstness denotes existence of all other properties such as function and change. In biology and physiology, it refers to protoplasmic structure on which all other properties depend. Any kind of function then depends on the lability of protoplasmic change, which permits the existence of secondary coordinated changes. Thirdness refers to directed or purposeful change. Biological structure, as has been shown in preceding chapters, is characterized by configurational negative entropy or by configurational free energy, which leads to the characteristic properties of hydration energy, irritability, and responsiveness. Renewal of expended free energy or negative entropy depends on metabolic sources of intracellular and extracellular materials. These yield continuous supplies of negative entropy that originate in carbohydrates of vegetable origin. As explained in chapter 3, the ultimate sources of energy and entropy depend on the photosynthetic conversion of radiant sunlight in the green leaves of plants.

The quality of firstness in animal biology thus embraces the ontological existence of intracellular protoplasm throughout the entire animal and vegetable kingdom. This always contains morphologically structured water, associated with the property of free energy of hydration or dielectric energy. Protoplasm and its attendant irritability are therefore primary and synechistic. Function is qualified by its secondness, since it depends on *changes* of dielectric energy and irritability or responsiveness. In higher organisms, such as vertebrates and mammals, this may be attended by extensive redistributions of dielectric energy and tension throughout many complicated systems of cells, tissues, and anatomical structures.

Thus, the primary and secondary properties of morphology and function are synechistically 'held together' and well-ordered. When extension in time is continuous with function and behavior, we obtain the quality of 'thirdness' or purposeful directed behavior. In addition to the constraining conditions of synechism, this is motivated in human life by agapism (the pursuit of happiness), and by tychism (the dictates of chance, fortune, and liberty). The life of reason depends on the pursuit of happiness within the realms of freedom and necessity. This is the common basis of well-directed creative, intelligent behavior extended over a lifetime or over all generations.

Reason and Protoplasm

The foregoing considerations lead to the conclusion that human reason is bound together synechistically with numerous other qualities of 'thirdness'. These include all the time-dependent properties of 'secondness', as they are related to irritability and responsiveness, particularly in the brain, sense organs, and neuromuscular systems. When these are joined together synechistically with the time-dependent qualities of understanding, perception, conceptions, knowledge, and behavior, we arrive at the faculty of reason, which is necessary in the pursuit of happiness. The indispensable property of protoplasm, necessary for 'secondness' and 'thirdness' and for mature adult reason is that of dielectric energy, hydration energy, negative entropy, and irritability. This can be observed only in living protoplasm — never in inanimate mechanisms. The latter are indifferent with respect to agapism, hence also to organistic reason. Therefore, pure technology develops only according to the principles of 'anancism', or evolution by mechanical necessity. Thus, 'thirdness' is inaccessible in a perfectly mechanistic universe, which lacks the quality of 'firstness' inherent in human protoplasm.

The external physical universe, as *William James* pointed out, is inherently pluralistic. It reaches human consciousness through sense impressions that act on human protoplasm in billions of nerve endings and afferent sensory nerves. According to the principles of Gestalt psychology, these billions of impressions are organized and unified synechistically to form a coherent holistic impression which becomes the unitary basis of empirical experience. Thus, the source of all experience is the direct contact of protoplasm with the pluralistic external universe. According to *James*' radical empiricism, human knowledge and reason are thus based on unorganized impressions received by living protoplasm. Conceptual knowledge, thought, and philosophy are attained by the non-experimental processes of introspection that man has inherited as part of permanent human reason. This is a property of 'thirdness' that is permanently coexistent and bound together with time.

Conclusions

In the preceding pages, the fundamental precondition of human reason has been taken as the phylogenetic existence of human protoplasm. It would be difficult to doubt the absolute validity of this presupposition. To do so would be to accept the metaphysical proposition of 'solipsism', or the idea that the external world of things, objects, percepts, and thought is completely illusory, and existent only in the mind or imagination. This has always been found to be completely unacceptable to metaphysical doctrine. There are only two alternative propositions. The first is that human protoplasm has the property of 'firstness' and that 'thought' and 'reason' are aspects of 'thirdness'. The other alternative (the Cartesian principle of 'cogito') is that thought presupposes existence. Then thought is real, and a property of 'firstness'. Existence is thus a derivative aspect of 'thirdness'. In the present period of physicochemical thought, the position of atoms and other particles in space and time has been habitually conceived of as an aspect of 'firstness', and the existence of living matter as an aspect of 'thirdness'. *Peirce* was of the opposite opinion (chapter 8). He considered non-living matter to be a degraded form of life. Hence, the non-living universe was regarded as an object of human thought. The term for this way of thinking he called 'objective idealism'.

Thus, objective reality is characterized by 'thirdness' in relation to the 'firstness of human protoplasm'. Thus, of all sciences, anthropology is characterized by its 'firstness': the others have the quality of 'thirdness', and are creations of human reason. In order to avoid the fault of circularity, it is necessary to derive all the sciences from the firstness of human protoplasm in the brain, sense organs, and neuromuscular system. Thus, human anatomy, physiology, and chemical morphology can be regarded as the primary sciences.

Bibliography

Adams, H.: The education of Henry Adams (Modern Library, New York 1900).

Adams, H.: The tendency of history (Macmillan, New York 1919).

Adrian, E.H.: The effect of internal and external potassium concentration on the membrane potential of frog muscle. J. Physiol., Lond. *133:* 647–658 (1956).

Alexander, S.: Space, time and deity (Dover, New York 1960).

Appel, F. W. and Appel, E.M.: Intracranial variations in the weight of the human brain. Hum. Biol. *14:* 69–84 (1943).

Bailey, P. and Bonin, G. von: The isocortex of man (University of Illinois Press, Urbana 1951).

Baldwin, J.M.: Dictionary of philosophy and psychology (Finch Press, 1902).

Balint, M.: Thrills and regression (Hogarth Press, London 1959).

Benedict, F.G. and Cathcart, C.I.: Muscular work (Carnegie Institute, Washington 1913).

Bernard, C.: Leçons sur les phénomènes de la vie communs aux animaux et aux végétaux (Baillière, Paris 1878).

Bergson, H.: The creative mind (Wisdom Library, New York 1946).

Boltzmann, L.: Populäre Schriften (Leipzig 1905).

Bondareff, W.: Morphology of connective tissue ground substance with particular regard to fibrillogenesis and aging. Gerontologia *1:* 222–233 (1957).

Born, M.: Volumes and heats of hydration of ions. Hoppe-Seyler's Z. physiol. Chem. *1:* 45–48 (1920).

Born, M.: Natural philosophy of cause and chance (Oxford University Press, London 1948).

Bourlière, F.: The natural history of mammals (Knopf, New York 1953).

Bridgman, P.: The logic of modern physics (Macmillan, New York 1927).

Brodmann, E.: Neue Ergebnisse über die vergleichende histologische Lokalisations der Grosshirnrinde mit besonderer Berücksichtigung der Stirnhirns. Anat. Anz. (1912).

Brown, R.: Botanische Schriften (Ness von Essenbeck, Leipzig 1825).

Brown, C.G. and Sherrington, C.S.: On the irritability of a cortical point. Proc. R. Soc. B *85:* 250–277 (1912).

Bruce, D.M. and Marshall, J.M., jr.: Some ionic and bioelectric properties of the amoeba *Chaos chaos.* J. gen. Physiol. *49:* 131–178 (1965).

Brul, E.L. du: Evolution of the speech apparatus (Thomas, Springfield 1958).

Cannon, W.B.: The wisdom of the body (Norton, New York 1932).

Cantor, G.: Contributions to the founding of the theory of transfinite numbers. Part I. Math. Ann. *46:* 481–512 (1895).

Cantor, G.: Contributions to the theory of the founding of transfinite numbers. Part II. Math. Ann. *49:* 217–246 (1897).

Caratheodory, C.: Investigations of the fundamentals of thermodynamics. Math. Ann. *67:* 355–386 (1909).

Carnot, S.: Reflexions sur la puissance motrice du feu (Paris, 1824).

Carr, H.W.: Leibniz (Dover, New York 1960).

Catchpole, H.R. and Joseph, N.R.: Muscular work and athletic records; in *Nelson and Morehouse* Biomechanics IV (University Park Press, Baltimore 1974).

Chomsky, N.: Cartesian linguistics (Harper & Row, New York 1966).

Christiansen, J.J.; Hill, C.C., and Izatt, R.M.: Ion binding by synthetic macrocyclic compounds. Science *174:* 459–467 (1971).

Collingwood, E.G.: Essay on metaphysics (Regnery, Chicago 1938).

Darlington, C.D.: Evolution of man and society (Simon & Schuster, New York 1969).

Dickerson, J.W.T. and Widdowson, E.W.: Chemical change in skeletal muscle during development. Biochem. J. *74:* 247–257 (1960).

Donnan, F.G.: Theory of membrane equilibrium and membrane potential in the presence of a non-dialyzable electrolyte. J. Electrochem. *17:* 572–581 (1911).

Duhem: L'évolution de la mécanique (Paris 1891).

Ecanow, B.; Gold, B.E., and Tunkmann, F.: Application of physical chemistry principles to the study of anxiety and depression. Psychiatry psychom. *21:* 121–127 (1972–1973).

Ecanow, B. and Klavans, E.L.: in Physical chemical models of membranes in models of human neurological diseases; 1st ed. (Excerpta Medica, Amsterdam 1974).

Eddington, A.S.: The nature of the physical world (Macmillan, New York 1929).

Einstein, A.: (1905–1908): Investigations of the theory of the Brownian movement (transl. *A.B. Cowper*) (Methuen, London 1926).

Engel, M.B.; Joseph, N.R.; Laskin, D.M., and Catchpole, H.R.: Am. J. Physiol. *201:* 621 (1961).

Fenn, W.B.: Electrolytes in muscle. Physiol. Rev. *16:* 150–187 (1935).

Ferguson, J.: The use of chemical potentials as indices of toxicity. Proc. R. Soc. B *127:* 387–404 (1939).

Foster, Sir M.: Lectures on the history of physiology (Dover, New York 1970).

Frege, G.: What is a function? Translations from the philosophical works of Gottlob Frege (Philosophical Library, New York 1952).

Frey-Wyssling, A.: Submicroscopic morphology of protoplasm (Elsevier, Amsterdam 1953).

Fritsch, O. und Hitzig, E.: Über die elektrische Erregbarkeit des Grosshirns. Arch. Anat. Physiol. *32:* 171–230 (1870).

Gersh, I. and Catchpole, H.R.: The nature of ground substance of connective tissue. Perspect. Biol. Med. *3:* 292–342 (1960).

Gibbs, J.W. (1875): On the equilibrium of heterogeneous substances; in Collected works, vol. 1 (Longmans, Green, New York 1928).

Gibbs, J.W.: Elementary principles in statistical mechanics. Yale University (1901) (Longmans, Green, New York 1928).

Gilson, E.: The unity of philosophical experience (Scribner's, New York 1937).

Glisson, F.: Anatomia hepatica (Amsterdam 1650).

Godel, K.: The completeness of the axiom of the functional calculus of logic, in *van Heijevoort* From Frege to Godel (Harvard University Press, Cambridge 1967).

Goldschmidt, V.M.: Geochemical distribution of the elements. Skriften Norske Videnskaps Akad. (Oslo). J. Mat. Natur Kl. *8:* (1926).

Haller, A. von: On sensible and irritable parts of the body (Stockholm 1753).

Havet, J.: Contributions a l'étude des systèmes nerveux des actinies. *18:* 285–418 (1901).

Hazlewood, C.F. and Nicholls, H.L.: Changes in muscle sodium, potassium, chloride, water and voltage during maturation in the rat; an experimental and theoretical study. Johns Hopkins med. J. *125:* 619–633 (1969).

Head, H.: Speech and cerebral localization. Brain *46:* 355–528 (1923).

Helmholtz, H. von: Über die Erhaltung der Kräfte (Berlin 1847).

Helmholtz, H. von (1862): The sensations of tone as physiological foundation for the theory of music (Dover, New York 1954).

Henderson, L.J.: The fitness of the environment (Macmillan, New York 1908).

Henderson, L.J.: Blood, a study in general physiology (Yale University Press, New Haven 1928).

Hertwig, O. und Hertwig, H.: Das Nervensystem und die Sinnesorgane der Medusen (Vogel, Leipzig 1878).

Hill, A.V.: Living machinery (Bell, London 1944).

Hill, A.V.: The mechanics of voluntary muscle. Lancet *ii:* 947–951 (1951).

Hodgkin, A.L.: The ionic basis of electrical activity in nerve and muscle. Biol. Rev. *26:* 330–408 (1951).

Hofmeister, F.: Zur Lehre von der Wirkung der Salze. Arch. exp. Path. Pharmakol. *24:* 247–260 (1888).

Huxley, T.H.: The physical basis of life (lay sermon, 1868); quoted in *Hardy* Collected papers (Cambridge University Press, London 1936).

Huxley, T.H.: Man's place in nature (University of Michigan Press, Ann Arbor 1959).

Huxley, Sir J.: The wonderful world of life (Doubleday, Garden City 1969).

James, W.: Pragmatism (Longmans, Green, New York 1908).

James, W.: A pluralistic universe (Longmans, Green, New York 1909).

James, W.: Radical empiricism (Longmans, Green, New York 1912).

Jolly, W.A.: The time relations of the knee-jerk and simple reflexes. J. exp. Physiol. *4:* 67–87 (1910).

Joseph, N.R.: Interaction of amino acids and salts. I. Zinc chloride. J. biol. Chem. *111:* 479 (1935).

Joseph, N.R.: Interaction of amino acids and salts. II. Sodium chloride and thallous chloride. J. biol. Chem. *112:* 489 (1936).

Joseph, N.R.: Heterogeneous equilibrium of aqueous solutions. The activity coefficient and membrane potential in mixtures of gelatin and salts. J. biol. Chem. *116:* 233 (1938).

Joseph, N.R.: Dependence of electrolyte balance on growth and development of cells and tissues; in *Elden* A treatise on skin (Wiley, Chichester 1971a).

Joseph, N.R.: Physical chemistry of aging (Karger, Basel 1971b).

Joseph, N.R.: Comparative physical biology (Karger, Basel 1973).

Joule, J.P.: Scientific papers (London 1884–1887).

Katz, J.: Die mineralischen Bestandteile des Muskelfleisches. Pflüger's Arch. ges. Physiol. *61:* 1–85 (1895).

King, M.C. and Wilson, A.C.: Evolution of two levels in humans and chimpanzees. Science *188:* 107 (1975).

Koestler, A.: The ghost in the machine (Macmillan, New York 1967).

Kolliker, A.: Handbuch der Gewebelehre des Menschen (Leipzig 1885).

Laidler, K.J. and Pegis, C.: The influence of dielectric saturation on the thermodynamic properties of aqueous ions. Proc. R. Soc. A *221:* 80–92 (1957).

Levi-Strauss, C.: Totemism (Beacon, Boston 1963).

Levi-Strauss, C.: The savage mind (University of Chicago Press, Chicago 1970).

Locke, J.: in *Lamprecht* Selections (Scribner's, New York 1968).

Loeb, J.: Proteins and the theory of colloidal behavior (McGraw-Hill, New York 1924).

Lorenz, K.: Studies in animal and human behavior, vols. I and II (Harvard University Press, Cambridge 1970 and 1972).

Lovejoy, A.O.: The great chain of being (Harper & Row, New York 1960).

Lowry, C.H. and Hastings, A.B.: in *Lansing* Quantitative histochemical changes. Cowdry's problems of aging; 3rd ed. (Williams & Wilkins, Baltimore 1953).

Macallum, A.B.: The inorganic composition of the blood in vertebrates and in invertebrates and its origin. Proc. R. Soc. B *82:* 602–611 (1910).

Macallum, A.B.: The paleochemistry of the body fluids and tissues. Physiol. Rev. *14:* 133–159 (1926).

Mach, E.: Science of mechanics (Open Court, LaSalle 1942).

Mayer, J.R.: Bemerkungen über die Kräfte der unbelebten Natur. Justus Leibigs Ann. Chem. *42:* 233 (1842).

McCulloch, W.S. and Pfeiffer, J.: Of digital computers called brains. Sci. Mon. *69:* 368–376 (1949).

Merleau-Ponty, M.: Phenomenology of perception (Routledge & Kegan Paul, London 1962).

Meyerson, E.: Identity and reality (Dover, New York 1962).

Miller, D.C.: The science of musical sounds (Macmillan, New York 1916).

Minchin, E.A.: An introduction to the study of the protozoa (Arnold, London 1912).

Mohl, H. von: Grundzeichen der Anatomie und Physiologie der vegetalischen Zelle (Braunschweig 1871).

Morehouse, L.E. and Miller, A.T.: Physiology of exercise (Mosby, St. Louis 1967).

Mouret, G.: l'Entropie (Paris 1896).

Nastuk, W.I.: The electrical activity of the muscle membrane at the neuromuscular membrane. J. cell. comp. Physiol. *35:* 249–272 (1951).

Nastuk, W.I. and Hodgkin, A.L.: The electrical activity of single muscle fibers. J. cell. comp. Physiol. *35:* 39–73 (1951).

Nicholls, J..: The electricical potential of denervated skeletal muscle. J. Physiol., Lond. *131:* 1–12 (1956).

Oparin, A.I.: Origin of life (Macmillan, New York 1938).

Paget, Sir R.: Human speech (Kegan Paul, London 1963).

Pareto, V.: The mind and society (Harcourt Brace, New York 1935).

Parker, G.H.: The elementary nervous system (Lippincott, Philadelphia 1918).

Pauling, L.: The nature of the chemical bond (Cornell University Press, Ithaca 1944).

Pearl, R.: The rate of living (Knopf, New York 1928).

Peirce, C.S.: Deduction, induction and hypothesis. Popular Science Monthly, August (1878).

Peirce, C.S.: The structure of theories. The Monist (1891).

Peirce, C.S.: Man's glassy essence. The Monist (1892).

Peirce, C.S.: Evolutionary love. The Monist (1893).

Four essays in *C.S. Peirce:* The essential writings, edited by *Edward C. Moore.*

Peirce, C.S.: Philosophical writings, edited by *Justus Buchler* (Dover, New York 1955).

Penfield, W. and Rasmussen, T.: The cerebral cortex of man (Macmillan, New York 1950).

Penfield, W. and Roberts, C.: Speech and brain mechanisms (Princeton University Press, Princeton 1955).

Piaget, J.: Main trends in psychology (Harper & Row, New York 1970).

Poincaré, H.: Thermodynamique (Paris 1903).

Poincaré, H.: The value of science (Dover, New York 1946).

Purkinje, J.E.: Beobachtungen und Versuche zur Physiologie der Sinne (Berlin 1825).

Purkinje, J.E.: Symbolae ad ovi avium historium (Breslau 1825).

Robertson, J.D.: The inorganic composition of muscle. II. The abdominal flexor muscle of the lobster, *Nephrops norvegicus.* J. exp. Biol. *38:* 707–738 (1961).

Rosenhof, R.A. von: Monatliche Insektenbelistigungen (Nuremburg 1753).

Rothschild, Lord and Barnes, H.: The inorganic composition of the sea urchin egg. J. exp. Biol. *30:* 530–541 (1953).

Sarton, G.: History of science (Harvard University Press, Cambridge, Mass. 1952).

Schleiden, M.: Grundzüge der wissenschaftlichen Botanik (Leipzig 1842).

Schrodinger, E.: What is life? (Cambridge University Press, Cambridge 1944).

Schultze, M.: Das Protoplasma der Rhizopoda und der Pflanzenzelle. Ein Beitrag zur Theorie der Zelle (Engelmann, Leipzig 1863).

Schwann, T.: Mikroskopische Untersuchungen über die Übereinstimmung in der Struktur und dem Wachstum der Tiere und Pflanzen (Berlin 1839).

Shaw, J.: Ionic regulation of the muscle fibers of *Carcinus maenas*. J. exp. Biol. *35:* 385–396 (1958a).

Shaw, J.: Further studies of ionic regulation in the tissue fibers of Carcinus maenas. J. exp. Biol. *35:* 902–910 (1958b).

Shaw, J.: Osmoregulation in the muscle fibers of *Carcinus maenas*. J. exp. Biol. *35:* 920–929 (1958c).

Sherrington, C.S.: Observations on the scratch reflex in the spinal dog. J. Physiol., Lond. *34:* 1–50 (1906).

Sherrington, C.S.: The integrative action of the nervous system (Yale University Press, New Haven 1920).

Sicher, H. and Brul, E.L. du: Oral anatomy (Mosby, St. Louis 1970).

Simpson, G.G.: Tempo and mode in evolution (Harper & Row, New York 1965).

Smith, H.W.: From fish to philosopher (Little, Brown, Boston 1953).

Spaulding, E.G.: The new rationalism (New York 1918).

Spinoza, B. (1663): Ethics (Oxford University Press, London).

Starling, E.H.: The law of the heart (Linacre lecture, London 1918).

Stensen, N.: De musculis et glandulis (Copenhagen 1664).

Sullivan, J.W.N.: Beethoven, his spriritual development (Knopf, New York 1928).

Svedberg, T.: Colloid chemistry (Chemical catalog, New York 1928).

Thompson, d'Arcy W.: On growth and form (Macmillan, New York 1944).

Trautwein, W.; Zink, K. und Kayser, K.: Über Membran- und Actionpotentials einzelner Fasern des Warmblüterskeletmuskels. Pflügers Arch. ges. Physiol. *251:* 20–34 (1953).

Waldenreich, F.: The special form of the human skull in adaptation to the human gait. Z. Morph. Anthrop. *24* (1924).

Wheeler, W.M.: Emergent evolution (Norton, New York 1928).

Whitehead, A.N.: Introduction to mathematics (Holt, New York 1911).

Whitehead, A.N.: Science and the modern world (Macmillan, New York 1925).

Whitehead, A.N.: Process and reality (Macmillan, New York 1929).

Widdowson, E.W. and Dickerson, J.W.T.: Chemical composition of the body; in *Comar and Bonner* Mineral metabolism, vol. 2a (Academic Press, New York 1964).

Wiener, N.: Cybernetics (Technology Press, Cambridge 1948).

Subject Index